W9-BUK-451

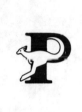

QUANTUM FITNESS

BREAKTHROUGH TO EXCELLENCE

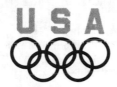

Irving Dardik, M.D., F.A.C.S.
Denis Waitley, Ph. D.

POCKET BOOKS
A DIVISION OF SIMON AND SCHUSTER
NEW YORK

Another *Original* Publication of POCKET BOOKS
Library of Congress Cataloging in Publication Data
Dardik, Irving.
Quantum fitness.

Bibliography: p.
1. Health.   2. Physical fitness.   3. Mind and body.
I. Waitley, Denis.   II. Title.
RA776.D218   1984   613.7   84-2165
ISBN 0-671-50903-9

POCKET BOOKS, A Division of Simon & Schuster, Inc.
1230 Avenue of the Americas, New York, N.Y. 10020
Copyright © 1984 by Denis Waitley, Inc. and Quantum Fitness Systems, Inc.

ISBN: 0-671-50903-9
First Pocket Books printing July, 1984
10 9 8 7 6 5 4 3 2 1

© Photographs by William Lulow
Fat-Cholesterol Chart, p. 186, © Reproduced with permission.
American Heart Association.

Jacket design by Milton Charles

We advise the reader to consult with his or her doctor before beginning
this, or any other regimen of diet and exercise. The authors and publisher
disclaim any liability, personal or otherwise, resulting from the proce-
dures in this book.

I dedicate this book to the Quantum future of
my children,
BELLE, SHIMONAH, ESTEE, and JUDAH.
And to ALISON, without whom this book would
not have been possible.

Irving Dardik

Dedicated to those individuals who dared to
excel, regardless of their background and circumstances.

Denis Waitley

We would like to thank the following corporations:

Amerec Corporation, PO Box 3825, Bellevue, WA 98009, provided us with the personal heart-rate monitoring system, the
Amerec 150 Sport Tester®* bicycle ergometers, rowing machines,
and their computerized treadmill.

Gravity Guidance, 1540 Flower Avenue, Duarte, CA 91010, the
originators of oscillating inversion equipment, provided us with
their research and their guiding system.

Procter & Gamble, Cincinnati, OH, made their Puritan Oil
brand scientific team available to us and provided research data on
cholesterol and polyunsaturated oils.

* Amerec 150 Sport Tester® is a trademark of Amerec Corporation, Bellevuw,
Washington.

ACKNOWLEDGMENTS

We owe our utmost appreciation to ALISON GODFREY, whose strength, vision and patience have been the driving force behind *Quantum Fitness*.

To MARGARET McBRIDE, our agent, we express our admiration for her ability to recognize new ideas and make them realities.

We would like to thank WILLIAM LULOW for his creativity in capturing the essence of exercise in photographs.

Our indebtedness also extends to MICHAEL WOLF, Ph.D., for his exceptional input, his quick thinking and his interpretive abilities in helping to structure this book.

Our whole-hearted thanks to RONALD BUSCH, president, and WILLIAM R. GROSE, editorial director of Pocket Books.

We appreciate the efforts of MILTON CHARLES, ANNE MAITLAND, ROGER BILHEIMER, MARCIA GABAY, KAREN WEITZMAN, JOHN GFELLER and the Pocket Books quantum sales force, and the Simon and Schuster production department.

And our special gratitude to our editor, SYDNY WEINBERG.

This book could not have been possible without our association with F. DON MILLER, Executive Director, United States Olympic Committee, and WILLIAM SIMON, President, United States Olympic Committee. Their commitment to excellence in sports and to the advancement of sports medicine has been an inspiration to our efforts.

Irving Dardik, M.D.
Denis Waitley, Ph.D.

CONTENTS

·

·

FOREWORD

I AM MOST pleased to contribute the foreword to *Quantum Fitness*, to share my personal enthusiasm for this book and to express my thoughts as to why I consider the concepts and ideals expressed herein so important to your personal fitness and health.

The Olympic motto, *Citius, Altius, Fortius* ("Swifter, Higher, Stronger"), clearly expresses the aspirations of athletes throughout the world as they reach out towards the heights of Olympic achievement. It was the ancient Greeks who established the Olympic Games with the understanding that excellence in performance demands a wholeness of body, mind and spirit. It is interesting to note that the modern science of quantum physics is reasserting this ancient Olympic ideal through its recognition that wholeness can only be realized within the *organization* of the elementary components of the universe. Similarly, new properties of wholeness arise as a result of the interaction and interconnection of the component elements which comprise athletic performance. And what better example than that of the Olympic rings? Seen in isolation a ring is simply a ring but when the five rings are properly interconnected, the message of the Olympic ideal is conveyed.

To introduce the latest scientific developments, and assist our athletes in their quest for excellence, the United States Olympic Committee has organized a Sports Medicine Council, chaired by Dr. Irving Dardik. In recognizing that strength and agility of the mind is critical for optimum strength and agility of the body, the Council has developed an outstanding psychology program headed by Dr. Denis Waitley.

The ideals of the Olympics are embodied in the concept of Quantum Fitness—the ability to be your absolute best, to reach and surpass goals you might not have thought were possible for you through the integration of body and mind. I am confident *Quantum Fitness* will make those concepts and techniques which are so important to the training and success of world class competitors available to all Americans.

F. Don Miller, Executive Director
United States Olympic Committee

QUANTUM FITNESS
AND YOU

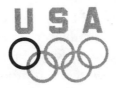

P REPARE YOURSELF. You are about to make a quantum leap to personal excellence.

According to quantum physics, the branch of science that orders the universe and studies the dynamic balance of changing and interacting systems, electrons do it all the time. Spinning around the nuclei of atoms, they leap from one level of energy to another, freeing even more energy in the process.

Like the invisible atom, you, too, are a microcosm of the universe, composed of many different systems. We are going to show you how to order your own mental and physical universe, bringing its key systems into a dynamic balance. It is this balance that will allow you to tap the limitless potential of individual energy that you alone possess. This Quantum connection will startle you both with its simplicity and the life changes it can create.

11

We are going to treat your mind and body as one system—an awesome, integrated, marvelously adaptable system. We are going to show you the connections between the sciences of psychology, nutrition and exercise, fusing them into a chain that will be far stronger than the sum of its individual links.

Like the ancient Greeks, the original Olympians who celebrated the integration of a healthy mind in a healthy body, our present-day Olympic athletes are in pursuit of perfection, seeking the moment when mind and body meld to propel them to a moment of world-class performance. In fact, this program began as an attempt to reduce the thousands of options available to our elite athletes and coaches to a structured, unified set of principles. These principles, which form the basis of the Quantum Fitness program, will work for you whether you're an armchair athlete or in pursuit of a gold medal.

The five chapters of this book fit together in five interlocking rings, like the symbol of the Olympic ideal. They represent the five continents of the world joining together in the spirit of cooperation and competition for the pure joy of the pursuit of excellence. The five Quantum rings represent the principles that, when applied to your own life, will create the energy to catapult you to Quantum Fitness.

THE QUANTUM CONNECTION

In the world of conventional science, the observer plays no part in the performance of the universe; it simply unfolds before him. In the world of quantum physics, however, the observer, by participation and experimentation, actually changes the nature and outcome of the performance. And in Quantum Fitness you participate in integrating the elements of your individual fitness program and create a new performance level for yourself.

Like a grand orchestra, the cosmos performs an everchanging symphony in perfect harmony. Everything in the universe is interconnected, from the limitless galaxies to the infinitesimal atom, and remarkably sensitive to the precise way in which the fundamental laws of physics manifest themselves. So delicate is the balance that the slightest shift in nature's orchestration would cause a cataclysmic change in the order of the universe.

The universe within you is even more marvelous. You have a brain capable of thinking at a rate of eight hundred words per minute, capable of replaying events from the past as if they were reoccurring and capable of envisioning events that have never happened as if they were actually occurring. Your body consists of more than ten thousand billion cells; your eyes have about one hundred million receptors; your ears contain more than twenty-four thousand fibers; your skeleton, which is composed of over two hundred bones, is the framework for six hundred plus muscles, over seven miles of nerve fiber and sixty thousand miles of blood vessels, which lead to a heart that pumps more than one thousand six hundred gallons of blood through them each day.

Disrupt the fragile balance within your body with negative thought patterns, poor nutritional habits and a sedentary life-style and the result may be disorder, disease and emotional discord.

Apply the dynamically balanced organization of the principles of Quantum Fitness and unlock your hidden potential to achieve the goals of good health, high performance and longevity.

YOU MAKE THE DIFFERENCE

The Quantum Fitness program treats your mind and body as an integrated system and identifies the connections between the many subsystems of which it is composed. It creates simplicity from complexity and identifies the principles that allow the most efficient and intelligent approach to fitness, which we define as good health, enhanced performance and longevity.

It is unique in that you don't have to try to measure up to someone else's idea of who you are or what you should achieve; there are no magic numbers that ignore your individuality. Although the Quantum program was inspired by our work with the Olympic athletes, it is designed for *you*—or, more accurately, it is designed *by* you. By applying the Quantum principles to your own needs, you can create your own short- and long-term fitness goals.

Quantum Fitness can be your program, regardless of your age, fitness level or current life-style. If you're already in great shape, terrific! Quantum Fitness can help you maintain your condition and will probably help you improve your performance. If you've lost some of the spring you once had in your step, and your belt is a little tighter than you'd like it to be, Quantum Fitness can put you back on the road to better habits and keep you there. And if you've only recently become concerned about improving the quality of your life, you've definitely come to the right place.

Even if you haven't been serious about fitness for years, there's hope for you. Researchers at Arizona State University and the University of Western Ontario tested formerly active individuals between the ages of thirty and thirty-nine. These people had not run, jogged, lifted a weight or been active in a fitness program in ten years or more. But once they participated in a program of physical activity three times a week for eight weeks, their endurance returned to high levels of fitness. *

THE QUANTUM FITNESS PLAN

Many fitness regimens today are easy to get into but even easier to get tired of, with single-idea approaches that can result in overtraining, undernourishment and even physical injury. Quantum Fitness, on the other hand, is the first approach to total well-being, and integrates the latest advances in exercise, nutrition and motivational technique. It is completely personalized; we give you the building blocks, but *you* are the architect of your individual program.

* Executive Fitness Newsletter, Rodale Press, Inc. Vol. 14, No. 14, July 9, 1983.

We will begin with the mind, the power we will call the Quantum Force. It is through the adaptive, responsive power of the mind that you will integrate the habits of good nutrition and sensible exercise into your life. We will show you how to employ what may already be a familiar concept to you, feedback, in tandem with a new one, feedforward, to tune into your body rhythms. You will learn to listen to your body speak to you through the window of your heartbeat, and use the information to tailor your own fitness goals.

Next we will explore Quantum Nutrition. Out of the hundreds of conflicting views on what to eat and how and when to eat it, we have distilled a simple, easy-to-understand and easy-to-follow diet program.

Then we introduce Quantum Exercise, a carefully organized and flexible program that will adapt and expand to meet your lifestyle and evolving fitness goals.

Finally, when you have achieved the dynamic balance of thought, nutrition and exercise, you will be ready to command the incredible hidden potential within you and make the Quantum leap.

THE QUANTUM PRINCIPLES

The term *dynamic balance* works on many levels. To the quantum physicist, it refers to the balance struck when entropy, the ultimate decay of all systems into chaos, is fought by the input of energy into the decaying system. To the civil engineer, it has a more easily grasped meaning: unless he continually maintains and rebuilds the bridges he has built (energy input), they will decay and collapse (entropy). On the level at which Quantum Fitness applies to you, it means an intelligent and carefully structured program of nutrients, mental and emotional choices and exercise that ensures optimal input of energy to brain and body to balance the processes of disease and aging (entropy).

15

As we wrote this book we were continually struck by the many ways in which dynamic balance must be sought. In Chapter Two it is the balance between positive and negative stress. In Chapter Three it is the balance of nutrients that must be consumed. In Chapter Four it is the alternation of exercise and recovery. And in all cases we see the three concepts that underlie and support the state of dynamic balance: *adaptation, variety,* and *rhythm.*

QUANTUM ACCESS CODES: THE KEYS TO THE QUANTUM PRINCIPLES

Each section of the Quantum program is ruled by a primary principle that governs but is not exclusive to that section. These principles connect the seemingly unrelated elements of the program, enabling you to adapt to environmental demands and directing your actions. The keys to applying these principles to your own life are the access codes, which form the basis for each section's core program.

Quantum Force

Primary Quantum principle: ADAPTATION.

Access codes: Adaptive Relaxation and simulation cycles.

Through the use of simple relaxation, visualization and self-talk techniques, you will learn to harness the Quantum Force of your mind to actualize your health, performance and longevity goals.

Quantum Nutrition

Primary Quantum principle: VARIETY.

Access codes: Fiber-based carbohydrates, lean-source protein and clear water.

By listening to your body's needs and supplying it with a selection of foods from the above-mentioned nutrient sources, you will maximize your energy and prepare your body for the benefits of Quantum Exercise.

Quantum Exercise

Primary Quantum principle: RHYTHM.

Access codes: Core balance, rhythmic endurance and multijoint patterning exercise.

These concepts will allow you to orchestrate an adaptive program that will work with the rhythm of *your* body, incorporating exercises for aerobic, anaerobic and flexibility benefits.

A NEW BEGINNING

As you read through this book you come to know and understand the dynamic balance of your personal universe within the cosmos. Using the Quantum Force, you will integrate the concepts of Quantum Nutrition and Exercise into your life, adjusting and adapting the program until it flows seamlessly into your daily routine.

At first the changes will be subtle, like the brush strokes that create shading and light on a painting, or the modulation of tempo and volume in a musical composition. Soon you will no longer be willing to follow the new fads in diet and exercise. You will have consciously, intelligently, chosen your own path, the right way for you alone. Breaking away from the pack, you will be ready to make the Quantum leap to excellence worthy of the world-class performer you are.

Positioned in the center of the fitness stage, you will be intimately connected to the rhythms of your mind and body, operating in complete harmony, with you as the conductor.

QUANTUM FORCE

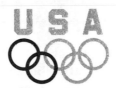

Y OUR MIND is the force behind Quantum Fitness; it is both the
lock on and the key to your door of success. Winners in
every walk of life have discovered that mental training is as important as physical training. Indeed, it is the critical edge of the
champion.

Many of the popular fitness programs we have analyzed concentrate on one particular physiological area of fitness. They
either emphasize exercise and add a nutritional garnish, or they
embellish a nutritional theme and suggest some exercise that may
be useful. If they mention the role of the mind at all, they refer
vaguely to some positive thinking and maybe add a soupçon of behavior modification as afterthoughts.

In our opinion the major reason that many members of our society are spectators rather than participants, and allow themselves

to be shuffled through the system, is because they lack an adequate understanding of the power of the human mind.

THE INNER WINNER

The air was thin and still on that October afternoon in 1968, and there was a hush of anticipation in the Olympic stadium. Bob Beamon had just leaped nearly thirty feet in the long jump, a record that remains unbroken as of this writing.

The attention of the 84,000 spectators at the Mexico City Olympics was now centered on the high jump bar, set at 2.24 meters (approximately 7 feet 4.2 inches), a record height. The athlete was a carrot-topped, freckle-faced youth by the name of Dick Fosbury, who had revolutionized the art of high jumping with the invention of a backward, headfirst dive known as the Fosbury Flop.

While the throng sat mutely, eyes glued to the bar, awaiting Fosbury's attempt, it intently studied Fosbury's prejump concentration. He stood about twenty yards directly in front of the bar, preparing for a straight-ahead running approach. His eyes were closed, his hands opened and closed rhythmically at his sides and he rocked back and forth, toe to heel. This ritual continued for nearly eight minutes.

The crowd began to murmur softly, becoming anxious, and the television commentator wondered aloud what was going on.

Then, with no warning, Fosbury broke into a lope that developed into a relaxed sprint. As he neared the bar he rotated his body 180 degrees on the way up, arched his back in a reverse swan dive and cleared the bar, which didn't even tremble, for a new world record.

Even more amazing than the feat of winning was Fosbury's own revelation of how he did it. In an interview after the competition we learned that Dick Fosbury, like so many other champions, was a master of visualization.

As Fosbury rocked back and forth with eyes closed he was mentally picturing every step to the bar—the push-off, the rotation, the back arch, the feet position—in advance. And when the mental rehearsal gave him a vivid picture of his success in clearing the bar, it was his signal that he was ready.

Visualization, or mental simulation, is not a new concept. We all have fantasized and acted out our "life scripts"—neurotic soap operas or magnificent epic movies—at some point in our lives. Some people may call this daydreaming, but in the case of a fifteen-year-old figure skater who kept falling down on the ice, these mental simulation techniques paid off quickly. Before the end of her stay at the Olympic Training Center, she was able to relax and mentally picture herself successfully completing a difficult jump that she had previously been unable to perform. Within weeks of her return home, she telephoned with the good news that she had completed the double axel on the ice too!*

During the past decade the techniques involved in visual imagery and mental rehearsal have grown from the oversimplified concepts of positive thinking to more scientific approaches that incorporate high-speed cinematography, digitized computer readouts and stop-action video replay and simulation technology.

The capability of your mind to preplay and replay performances as if they were really happening is the central theme in applying the Quantum principles to fitness.

Current neurological and psychological research seems to confirm the incredible ability of the mind to drive the body to achieve the individual's immediate dominant thought by instructing the body to carry out the vivid images of performance as if they had been achieved before and are merely being repeated.

With preplay simulation (or feedforward) you can engrave in your mind the verbal, visual and emotional conditions associated with high performance, good health and long life. This process greatly influences your daily habit patterns and acts as a steering

* May, Jerry, Ph.D. *Clinics in Sports Medicine*, Vol. 2, No. I, pg. 96, March, 1983.

program toward your goals. With replay simulation (or feedback) you can replay your successes during quiet times or off days to reinforce your self-confidence in your fitness progress. The feedback also allows you to enter new, positive, corrective data into your thoughts so that you can reset your aim on goals that were previously missed.

Winners see the act of winning before it ever happens. They act like winners, imagining with words, pictures and feelings the roles they want to play. When they make errors, miss or lose, they view failure as corrective feedback to help them hit their target next time. They give themselves a preview of coming attractions, and their coming attractions are usually the rewards of success rather than the penalties of failure. What you see in your mind's eye is what you get!

THE UNLIMITED SOURCE WITHIN

It's one thing to know that you can program yourself for success, and another, almost impossible task to understand how and why. The brain is hopelessly complex; all human inventions, including the Xerox machine, the camera, the microchip, the lunar excursion module, the electron microscope and the video tape recorder are toys by comparison. Biologist Lyall Watson pretty well sums it up: "If the brain were so simple that we could understand it, *we* would be so simple we couldn't!"

We are only just beginning to discover the virtually limitless capacities of the mind, and we've learned more about how the brain functions during the past decade than in all of our previous years of human existence. The Brain Research Institute at the University of California at Los Angeles has concluded that the ultimate creative capacity of the human brain may be infinite. That means the only limits it has are the ones you set yourself.

To take the Quantum leap into total fitness, you will need to understand a few critical concepts of how your brain functions.

THE QUANTUM CONNECTION BETWEEN THINKING AND FEELING

Your brain is divided into two major components: the *cerebral cortex* or upper part of the brain, and the *subcortex*, or lower part. The subcortical areas of the brain house your feelings and emotions. They compose the basic control center for the autonomic body functions, such as breathing, heart rate, blood-vessel diameters and body-temperature, functions that were for years considered involuntary. Today we know that we can exert conscious control over these functions through the use of biofeedback, relaxation and certain imagery techniques.

The cerebral cortex houses your higher-order thinking or intelligence functions, such as language, memory and judgment. This bulging mass of nervous tissue is what we generally see when the brain is pictured. It is divided into two hemispheres, the left and the right. Most researchers now concur that the left hemisphere, which controls the right side of the body, contains many of the verbal, logical and analytical functions. The right hemisphere, which controls the left side of the body, functions as the visual, intuitive and holistic partner.

Radiating upward from your brain stem is a small network of cells, about four inches in length, called the reticular activating system. It is just about the size and shape of a quarter of an apple, and is one of the most important parts of your body—and your mind—for you to understand and utilize to reach your Quantum goals.

This is literally the Quantum connection, the bridge between mind and body that makes thinking and feeling inseparable. It is the fiber you will use to bind your mind into your nutrition and exercise program and create a harmonious symphony out of all the variables in your life.

The reticular core of the brain dominates your behavior patterns, which include your eating habits, exercise habits and the

23

way you choose to live your life. It is perfectly placed to monitor all of the nerves connecting the brain and the body, and it "knows" what is going on better than any other single part of the brain. It can override activity in the spinal cord; it regulates the signals from the eyes, ears and other sense organs and is clearly linked to the display and feeling of emotions.

The reticular activating system performs the unique function of filtering incoming stimuli, such as sight, sound and touch, and deciding what information is going to become part of your experience. It decides what is important information and what is to be ignored. For example, if you live along a busy street, the reticular activating system quickly allows you to tune out the sound of cars rushing by.

Once you have made a decision that a certain value, thought, feeling, sound or picture is significant to you, your reticular activating system is alerted and it immediately transmits to your consciousness any information it receives regarding that item. So when you buy a new car, it is this network that suddenly causes you to notice all the cars of the same make—or even the same color—on the highway.

The beautiful feature about your reticular system is that you can program it to be on the alert for success-related input. It will wake you up in the morning without an alarm clock. If it knows you want the best nutrition program, it will home in on those foods you have identified as important to eat. It will help push you away from the table before you reach for seconds. It will remind you that it's time to jog, go to jazzercise class or take a walk. It explains why some people see a problem in every solution—and why *you* look for the solution in every problem.

While the reticular activating system is a physical part of the brain, the corresponding *self-image* is an abstract part of the brain, a function of the mind. And your self-image is the "habit thermostat" that sets the limits and the ceiling on your performance in your world.

YOUR AUTOMATIC PILOT TO FITNESS

Every living organism has a built-in autopilot to help it achieve its goal, which is, in very basic terms, to live. In more primitive forms of life, *to live* simply means physical survival for both the individual and the species. This built-in mechanism or instinct in animals is limited to finding food and shelter, avoiding or overcoming enemies and procreation to ensure the continuation of the line.

Humans have intelligence and emotional and spiritual needs and capabilities, which animals do not have, and we often overlook the fact that human beings have a success instinct. Animals cannot select their goals; their success mechanisms are limited to those inborn goal images that are called instincts. The success instinct in the human being, however, has something that animals will never possess: the creative imagination. The human being is the only creature on the earth that can direct his or her future by choice. You are more than a creature; you are a creator. You choose what your reticular activating system in your brain gives credit to. And you choose what you are looking for in the future through the repeated use of your creative imagination. The way you perceive your world defines the world in which you live. To see it in its unlimited range of possibilities is to see with the Quantum mind.

The perceptions we hold of ourselves, or our self-images, determine the kind and scope of people we are; our self-images are our life-controlling mechanisms and dwell at the subconscious level of thinking. Responsible for autonomic body control, such as breathing and heartbeat, and also for storing conditioned reflexes (repeated skills or images), the subconscious can be compared to a navigational guidance system or automatic pilot. The conscious level of thinking, responsible for collecting information from the environment, storing it in the memory and making rational decisions, can be compared to an attorney or judge.

Guidance systems can be programmed to seek an image or target. They are installed in missiles and spacecraft, which are then guided by these highly sophisticated electronic systems to seek a target through the use of electronic data feedback. The homing torpedo, for example, is a self-propelled system that makes every correction necessary to stay on target and score a hit by constantly monitoring feedback signals from the target area and adjusting the course setting in its own navigational guidance computer. Programmed incompletely or nonspecifically, or aimed at a target too far out of range, the homing torpedo will wander erratically until its propulsion system fails or it self-destructs.

So it is with each of us. Set a goal or an image and this self-motivated system, which constantly monitors self-talk and environmental feedback about the goal, adjusts the self-image settings in our minds and makes every decision necessary to reach the goal.

Most of the information fed into your subconscious memory stays there. The billions of separate bits of input stored over a lifetime are all there awaiting retrieval, and can never be willfully erased by you. They can be overridden or modified over a period of time, but you are stuck with them for life. While performing brain surgery on patients who were conscious under local anesthesia, Dr. Wilder Penfield of the Montreal Neurological Institute stimulated certain brain cells with a weak electrical current. Incredibly, he found his patients remembering experiences that had happened to them many years before; it was as if each person had a videotape recorder in his or her head. One thirty-five-year-old woman recalled her fifth birthday party in vivid detail. She saw all the children around her in party hats; she saw herself opening her presents, including a Dutch doll with wooden shoes, and she blew out the candles on her cake and made a wish. On the basis of this work, Dr. Penfield theorized that every experience, sight, sound, smell, taste and touch registers a pattern in the brain that stays long after the actual experience is consciously forgotten.

Recent research suggests that the brain can function like a holographic projector, which uses laser beams to project and reassemble three-dimensional images. If you've been through the delightful experiences of Disneyland, Walt Disney World or Epcot Center, you've been startled and amazed at the "real-life" ghosts and characters. Though they are just an assembly of light waves, they appear so solid that you could reach out and touch them! It is this holographic capability of the brain that makes your mind such a potent force in the Quantum program.

Scientists agree that the human nervous system cannot tell the difference between an actual experience and one imagined vividly, emotionally and in detail. Many of your everyday decisions are based upon information about yourself that has been stored as truth but is just a figment of your imagination, shaded by your environment.

During every moment of our lives, we program our self-image to work for us or against us. It strives to meet the objectives we set for it, regardless of whether they are positive or negative, true or false or safe or dangerous. Like a videotape recorder playing its cassette, its sole function is to follow instructions implicitly, based upon previous inputs.

THE CHILD IN YOUR PAST

The creative development of your self-image is one of the keys to developing Quantum Fitness. By the time we're thirty, each of us carries around with us a mental videotape cassette containing some three trillion pictures and holograms of ourselves in action. We may be vaguely conscious of its existence or we may not recognize it at all. But it is there.

These self-images are our own conceptions, or holograms, of the sorts of people we are, built by our own beliefs about ourselves. Most of these beliefs about ourselves have been unconsciously formed from our past experiences, our successes and failures, our humiliations, our triumphs and the way other people have reacted to us, especially in early childhood. Once ideas or beliefs about ourselves go into our self-images, they become true as far as we are concerned. We do not question the validity of these pictures, but act upon them as if they were true.

As we were growing up, many of us played an inferior role to the adults in our lives. We were told what to do and what not to do. We were constantly reminded of our shortcomings: "When I was your age I was already earning my own spending money." "Why couldn't you get straight *A*'s?" "Why are you so clumsy?" "Can't you do anything right?"

A child's self-image is very pliable and susceptible to external pressure and criticism, and this bombardment of negative feedback can take a toll. For example, young students who are treated by teachers and parents as though they are mentally slow will assume they are inferior to other children and behave accordingly.

Low achievers water and cultivate the early seeds of inferior feelings with their imaginations; these feelings grow and multiply like strong, prickly weeds and will stick and irritate them for years to come.

BEAUTY AND THE BEST

Unfortunately, in our society, the idea of beauty is still largely based on external characteristics. The ideal woman has the youth of Brooke Shields, the photogenic appeal of Christie Brinkley, the endurance of Mary Decker and the ever-trim figure of Jane Fonda. Her male counterpart is a combination of Tom Selleck, O. J. Simpson, Cary Grant and Michael Jackson, served up in an NFL warm-up suit.

As we become more concerned with appearances and immediate sensual gratification, there is an increasing number of people who will go to any extreme to look young and beautiful and to achieve fame and fortune. When we look in the mirror after starving ourselves on four hundred calories a day for three weeks and training for the marathon after an hour's worth of aerobics, we see ourselves as inadequate compared to our television and motion-picture idols. So we give up any attempt at fitness because the standards we used to measure our progress were external ones and therefore unrealistic.

Most people tend to be either apathetic or cynical about personal development. On the one hand they know that knowledge and effort bring about change, but on the other hand they resist that change. They realize that many people have struggled to greatness and overcome enormous obstacles to become successful, but they can't imagine that it can happen to them. These low achievers learn the habit of concentrating on their failures, so they resign themselves to be the also rans, wishing and envying away their lives. Because they are controlled by external standards set by others, they often set their sights too high and are unrealistic to begin with, and as they fail to reach their goals again and again, these failures become set in their subconscious self-images. This is why so many people have "permanent potential." In other words, they *almost* succeed over and over, but these short-lived successes fail to materialize into solid achievements.

But you are a Quantum individual. To you, beauty radiates from the inside out. You have a deep-down-inside feeling of your own worth. You want to fit in, take part and earn the respect of others, but you do not conform to the external standards of the group. Recognizing your uniqueness, you develop and maintain your own high standards that will make you the best you can be.

You accept yourself as you are right now—an imperfect, changing, growing and worthwhile person. And you are eager to learn the Olympic techniques of fitness.

A MAJOR QUANTUM ACCESS CODE: ADAPTIVE RELAXATION

In Chapter One we referred to the keys to dynamic balance in the Quantum Fitness program called Quantum Access Codes. The first of these codes is adaptive relaxation. Much of our knowledge on this subject is associated with the late Dr. Hans Selye, the acknowledged father of stress research. Dr. Selye's definition of stress, now nearly fifty years old, is still one of the best we've encountered: "Stress is the body's nonspecific response to any demand placed on it, whether that demand is pleasant or not."

Is stress good or bad? It depends on how you look at it. Dr. Selye observed that sitting in a dentist's chair or kissing passionately can be equally stressful, although not necessarily equally agreeable. Good stress, or eustress, associated with feelings of desire, volition and reward, leads to goal orientation, energy, power and a sense of well-being. Bad stress, or distress, which is associated with feelings of fear, compulsion and inhibition, leads to confusion, dysfunction and disease.

At the first hint of a dangerous or threatening confrontation from the environment, the body automatically musters its defenses in preparation for fight or flight. Today, instead of a saber-toothed tiger or a cave bear pursuing us, it's a Honda Civic in front of us or a highway patrol car behind us that stirs up the juices. As our blood pressures jump, our heart rates quicken, our arteries constrict and the adrenaline pumps, we rush headlong into an imaginary struggle for survival. This kind of daily frustration is called invisible entrapment, and to compensate we tend to drink more, smoke more, and fret more to cope or escape.

The antianxiety drugs, increasing in use in the United States today (over sixty-five million tablets consumed annually), serve to reduce emotional reactions to threats of pain or failure. But unfortunately they also interfere with the ability to learn to tolerate these stresses. It is far better to develop behavioral methods of coping with one's problems than to try to dissolve them with a pill.

According to Dr. Selye, all of us have a "stress savings account" deposited in our bodies as energy, or our life force. The object is to use it wisely over the longest time span possible. The difference between our stress savings account and a normal bank account is that we cannot make any more deposits in our life force; we can

only make withdrawals. The reason most people age at such different rates is that our society is full of "big spenders" (the so-called
Type A personalities) who overreact to harmless circumstances as
if they were life-or-death matters.

Adaptability is the key in a changing universe. By anticipating
the probable action of others through empathy and by remaining
open and receptive to change, we need not allow others to ruin
our days with their bad days. In most of our daily confrontations,
hostility and anger can be dealt with by relaxation and exercise.

Adaptive relaxation helps relieve the distresses of life, which
can lead to major health problems such as heart attacks, strokes,
high blood pressure and gastrointestinal disorders. It helps us cope
with frustration and anxiety, leaving us more energy for positive
pursuits. It relieves fatigue and allows us to sleep better. It can
even reduce the tendency to smoke, compulsive eating, alcohol
dependency and drug abuse.

In the Quantum Fitness program we use adaptive relaxation,
not only to relieve physical and emotional tension and distress, but
to place the mind and body in the most receptive state for feedforward simulation in advance, maximum achievement during
performance and feedback reinforcement after performance.

One of the best and most successful adaptive relaxation techniques is autogenic training, developed by the German psychiatrist Johannes H. Schultz in 1932. The word *autogenic* comes from
the Greek combining forms *auto-*, meaning self-, and *-genic*,
meaning being born or being productive. It is translated to mean
"selfproductive."

The West Germans, East Germans, Soviets and other Eastern
European countries have used autogenic training in their elite and
Olympic athlete programs for many years. Although there are
many different types of relaxation techniques that are equally effective, we recommend autogenic training in the Quantum Fitness
program because it is very restful and teaches "passive concentration," which allows the mind and body to self-regulate toward a

more harmonious state. Autogenic relaxation training also maximizes the receptivity of the mind for visualization and self-talk simulations, and is the ideal progression toward biofeedback training.

Autogenic Training Exercises

Before you begin:

Find a quiet place, where there will be no noise or interruptions for at least twenty minutes. The most convenient position may be reclining in a comfortable chair with a good back rest, or lying flat on a bed or carpeted floor with your arms at your sides and your feet a few inches apart and pointed slightly away from you. If you have a tendency to fall asleep during relaxation training, you may want to sit in a straight-backed chair. If you're sitting, let your head fall and relax gently forward, feet apart on the floor, back straight, arms bent and resting apart in your lap or at your sides. It's important to keep your eyes closed once you begin the exercises, to help you block any external stimulation that may interrupt your passive concentration. You'll find it easy to realize the optimal benefits of these exercises by silently repeating sentences to yourself over and over again without trying to force the results to happen. The less you try to force these exercises, the more effective they'll be. In autogenic training, relaxation is the key. The autogenic training exercises consist of six very simple sentences, which are going to be said repeatedly. Pay attention to the sentences as you say them, and let each sentence have its effect and impact on your body. Once you learn the six sentences, close your eyes, breath deeply and begin the exercise.

The First Exercise Involves the Concept of Heaviness. Start with the right arm if you are right-handed.

My right arm is heavy. I'm at peace. My right arm is heavy. My right arm is heavy. I'm relaxing. My right arm is heavy. My left arm is heavy. I'm relaxing. My left arm is heavy. My left arm is heavy. I'm at peace. My left arm is heavy. Both of my arms are heavy. Both of my arms are heavy. Both of my arms are heavy, Both of my arms are heavy.

My right leg is heavy. I'm at peace. My right leg is heavy. My right leg is heavy. I'm relaxing. My right leg is heavy. My left leg is heavy. I'm relaxing. My left leg is heavy. My left leg is heavy. I'm at peace. My left leg is heavy. Both of my legs are heavy. Both of my legs are heavy. Both of my legs are heavy. Both of my legs are heavy.

My arms and legs are heavy. My arms and legs are heavy. My arms and legs are heavy. My arms and legs are heavy.

The key for this heaviness exercise is *My arms and legs are heavy.*

The Second Exercise Focuses on the Sensation of Heaviness and Warmth.

My right arm is heavy and warm. I'm at peace. My right arm is heavy and warm. My right arm is heavy and warm. I'm relaxing. My right arm is heavy and warm. My left arm is heavy and warm. I'm relaxing. My left arm is heavy and warm. My left arm is heavy and warm. I'm at peace. My left arm is heavy and warm. Both of my arms are heavy and warm. Both of my arms are heavy and warm. Both of my arms are heavy and warm. Both of my arms are heavy and warm.

The key sentence for this exercise is *My arms and legs are heavy and warm.*

The Third Exercise Focuses on the Heart Rate.

My heartbeat is calm and regular. My heartbeat is calm and regular. My heartbeat is calm and regular. My heartbeat is calm and regular. My heartbeat is calm and regular. My heartbeat is calm and regular. My heartbeat is calm and regular. My heartbeat is calm and regular.

The key sentence for this exercise is *My heartbeat is calm and regular.*

The Fourth Exercise Focuses on Respiration, Allowing the Body to Breathe by Itself.

My breathing is relaxed and effortless. My breathing is relaxed and effortless. My breathing is relaxed and effortless. My breathing is relaxed and effortless. My breathing is relaxed and effortless. My breathing is relaxed and effortless. My breathing is relaxed and effortless. My breathing is relaxed and effortless.

The key sentence is *My breathing is relaxed and effortless.*

The Fifth Exercise Focuses on Warmth in the Abdominal Area.

My stomach is warm. My stomach is warm. My stomach is warm. My stomach is warm. My stomach is warm. My stomach is warm. My stomach is warm. My stomach is warm.

The key sentence is *My stomach is warm.*

The Sixth Exercise Focuses on Cooling of the Forehead.

My forehead is cool. My forehead is cool. My forehead is cool. My forehead is cool. My forehead is cool. My forehead is cool. My forehead is cool. My forehead is cool.

The key phrase for this exercise is *My forehead is cool.*

As you are doing the relaxation exercises, take a moment to think about the state they put you in. Compare the feelings your body produces during the exercises with the ones it produced before you began. With practice you will begin to bring about this relaxed state in a shorter period of time and will be able to maintain the state for a longer period of time.

As you complete the last of the six exercises, keep your eyes closed and extend your arms out in front of you. Take a deep breath in, flex your arms and slowly let your breath out. As you let it out, let your arms relax and open your eyes. You will feel wide awake, refreshed and alert but very relaxed.

If you decide to tape-record the autogenic training exercises in your own voice (which we highly recommend), say each phrase slowly and softly, pausing for about two seconds between each phrase. It may be helpful to play music in the background as you record the verbal exercises. We suggest classical music by Bach, Handel, Vivaldi or other artists from the baroque era, with a slow tempo in four-quarter time (about one beat per second) to heighten the effect. The music should be slightly stronger than your voice, but not overpowering, or distracting.*

After four to six weeks of daily practice you should be able to create the autogenic condition in just a few minutes, without the repetitions or the tape, by simply sitting quietly and remembering the phrases and the previous feelings from the practice sessions. This mental adjustment is very helpful before an event that requires your peak performance or during a crisis of any kind.

VISUALIZATION

As you learned at the beginning of this chapter, Olympic champions like Dick Fosbury have mastered the art of visualization in sports. Skiers, ice skaters, runners, gymnasts, weight lifters, fencers, volleyball players, archers and equestrian performers all credit visualization as a major factor in their success.

Visualization is not reserved for athletes only. Sales executives, pilots, dancers, musicians, actors, parents, hostesses, chefs, engineers, lovers and students do it every day.

Visualization can also be used to improve health and well-being. Dr. Gerald Jampolsky, a well-known psychiatrist from California, has had a great deal of success using "healing visualization" with

* Information on prerecorded autogenic-exercise audio tapes may be obtained by writing to Autogenic Tapes, Box 197, Rancho Santa Fe, CA, 92067.

both children and adults. He also uses visualization to help students with learning disabilities.

In a typical group session Dr. Jampolsky tells his young patients to put away their "thinking minds" and put on their "seeing minds." He then instructs them to create a mental blackboard, complete with chalk and eraser. Anytime a child sees words or phrases such as *can't, impossible, ought to, should,* and *if only* on the blackboard, he or she is instructed to mentally erase those words or phrases. Dr. Jampolsky then has the children think about their disease and try to imagine what it looks like. He helps them understand what it actually looks like in their bodies. He then helps the children form positive mental pictures of their disease receding and of themselves recovering. Obviously this technique is a supplement to and not a replacement for traditional medical treatment.

Perhaps the most dramatic work in visualization techniques to improve health is being done by Drs. Carl and Stephanie Simonton in Texas. The Simontons are using visualization, along with traditional medical therapy, to treat seriously ill cancer patients. The Simontons' approach is to get the patient to accept the responsibility for his or her illness and its cure; then they teach him or her to utilize deep relaxation and visualization exercises. One basic technique is to see the cancer and then imagine an army of healthy white blood cells attacking it and carrying off the diseased cells. The patient sees him- or herself becoming totally healthy again. The Simontons have had an impressive number of case histories of people who have experienced complete remission from supposedly incurable cancer after using their visualization methods.

But maybe you're saying to yourself right now, "Wait a minute, I didn't buy this book to help me overcome cancer; I'm reading it to learn how to win more in my everyday life!" Bear with us. Whether you are an elite athlete, or slightly overweight, or just get a little winded when you get out of your golf cart for your next shot, visualization is for you too!

Visualization works because the mind reacts automatically to the information we feed it in the form of words, pictures and emotions. Remember, the mind cannot tell the difference between an imagined experience and a real one, and therefore responds to what you think or imagine to be true. The act of vividly imagining a scene in your mind makes it a real experience.

Basically there are two types of visualization, programmed and receptive. Programmed visualization is used to get what we want out of life. We picture what we want repeatedly and the brain sends signals to the body that cause us to take action to bring about the desired results.

To reach your Quantum goals, you need to be specific in exactly what you want. For example, see yourself in a bathing suit and weighing 125 pounds. See yourself eating specific portions of certain foods. Feel your pulse at a certain rate during aerobic exercise, and then feel it return to your normal rate within a specified period of time.

It is better to visualize your goals in increments, just out of reach but not out of sight. Visualize conditions and things that are consistent with your personal and moral values. If there is a conflict, you will be less likely to achieve what you want. Ask yourself if what you are picturing is in your own best interests and in the best interests of those who will be affected. Make sure you really want what you are visualizing; *never* picture a condition or event you don't want to occur.

And, most important, when you visualize yourself, see yourself in the present, as if you are already accomplishing one of your goals. Make certain your visual image is as you would see it through your own eyes, not watching through the eyes of a spectator.

One middle-aged woman to whom we had taught these principles decided to use them to change some aspects of her life. She had not worked outside her home since her children were born, but now that they were all in school, she longed for some outside activity to enrich her days. In the process of devoting herself to her family, she had allowed herself to become overweight and had lost much of her self-confidence.

After learning a relaxation technique that was comfortable for her, she began practicing visualization. She saw herself as a slim, trim 125 pounds and pictured herself looking lovely in a new dress and a new suit with a high-necked blouse with ruffled sleeves. She felt her self-confidence beginning to return as she mentally rehearsed seeking employment and interviewing for jobs. She saw herself smiling and relaxed during the interviews, and practiced the way she would answer the interviewer's questions.

Within four months this determined lady dropped from 165 to 125 pounds and found a part-time position with flexible hours that allowed her to fulfill her professional needs yet be at home when her children returned from school. She is now a self-assured, radiant woman whose personality shines in all the facets of her life.

Receptive visualization is used to help answer a question or find a solution to a problem. In this type of visualization the question is formulated or the problem posed. First the issue is analyzed logically for better understanding; then a mental picture of a blank screen is formed, and the answer or solution is allowed to appear on the screen in its own time. This technique is especially helpful in recalling information that appears to have been forgotten or lost.

To enhance your ability to visualize better, learn really to be in the present, mentally as well as physically. Start taking mental notes of all the worthwhile sensual experiences in your life. Take in as many sights, sounds, smells, textures and tastes as you can. Watch the beauty of a sunrise or sunset. Feel the wet sand of a beach between your toes. Feel the coolness of the evening breeze on your face. Listen to the sounds and smell the newly mowed hay as you drive through the country. Reach out and physically touch those around you more often. Be more curious about *everything* around you.

Another specific way to improve your visualization skills is to use them more in your everyday conversation. As you listen to someone talk, try to form a mental image of the situation he or she describes. Allow the words to form images, feelings and sensations. When you talk to others, use words that are rich in visual imagery; word pictures, analogies, stories, metaphors and similes create vivid mental pictures. You will enjoy a side benefit of becoming a better conversationalist and public speaker if you do.

As you learn to become more observant you will find your powers of visualization improving. Reminisce about a pleasant vacation you have had. Close your eyes and let your attention drift back to that time. Recall the feelings you had at the time and relive them as you allow the images to come into your mind. By linking feelings and images, you will be able to recall both better. Say with your mental voice the names of some of the places you visited. Now focus on one especially memorable part of one of the experiences. Remember how it looked to you, what you heard, how you felt and what you did. Relive the episode in your imagination as vividly as possible. Go ahead: Stop reading this book, close your eyes and go back to a special place in space and time.

Isn't that a great turn-on? That is the power of the mind—that amazing ability to replay in vivid detail the remembrance of things past.

Visualization Exercises

Go to a quiet place, with no distractions, and put yourself into a state of deep relaxation. You may use the autogenic training exercises referred to in this chapter, or you may already have your own method. Use your own technique if it works for you. Remember, the key to Quantum Fitness is that *you* make the difference. When you are relaxed, take yourself on a trip in the country.

See yourself walking down a long, winding country road toward a big red barn. Observe the shape of the barn as you get closer, and notice the intensity of its color. Examine the entire building. Is it a large or small barn? What do the doors look like? The windows?

As you approach the barn, run your hand across the side of it, feeling the texture of the wood. Is it rough or smooth? Do you feel any splinters? Is it painted or stained?

Now open the door and go inside. Do you see any animals? Look at all the different objects in the barn. Notice their colors, shapes and sizes. Do you see any hay? Is there a hayloft? Are there any tools and equipment? Take a deep breath and notice the smells of the barn. Are they pleasant or unpleasant? Take a final look around and then walk back outside and close the door.

As you move away from the barn you notice a grassy area that has beautiful wild flowers growing in it. You walk toward this area, taking in the fragrance of the flowers and noticing their bright colors. What colors are they? On the grassy area you reach down and pull off your shoes and socks and run your bare feet through the cool dampness of the grass. You lie down on the grass, and for a moment you bury your head in the thick, tall grass, just like you did when you played hide-and-seek as a kid. Smell the fresh scent of the grass and the flowers.

Now roll over on your back and look up into the sky. What shapes are the clouds? Which way are they moving? Suddenly a hawk darts into your view and dives,with wings slightly folded, toward the ground. The hawk realizes it is pursuing a false target and swoops gracefully skyward again and begins to circle higher and higher. As you lie there you notice the warmth of the sun on your face. You soak it in for a few moments and reflect on how good you feel. You feel completely relaxed and at peace. You can come here at any time in your imagination and that pleases you.

Now you allow yourself to come back gently. Become aware of your position, your surroundings and your body. Feel the sensation in your toes, legs, body, arms and head. Stretch your arms in front of you, open your eyes and notice the calm aura that surrounds you.

This process develops your inner senses. You can practice by visualizing any place that you would like to visit in your mind.

Continual practice will help you really "see" the sights, "hear" the sounds, "smell" the smells and "feel" the surroundings.

Let's try another exercise. Again, get in a comfortable position and relax, breathing deeply. Concentrate on the feeling of calmness and serenity as you relax and let go. Using your inner senses of sight, sound, taste, touch and smell, visualize the following:

A picture of the house or houses you grew up in . . .
The face of a loved one . . .
The way your bedroom looks . . .
Your own reflection in a full length mirror . . .
A football game on television . . .
The sound of a train in the distance . . .
. . . of children laughing and playing . . .
. . . of waves lapping on the beach . . .
The feel of soft covers . . .
. . . of an itch on your back . . .
. . . of warm sunshine on your face . . .
The taste of a juicy orange . . .
. . . of a pretzel . . .
. . . of toothpaste . . .
. . . of a dill pickle . . .
The smell of newly cut grass . . .
. . . of a locker room . . .
. . . of freshly baked pie . . .
The feeling of hunger . . .
. . . of an exciting accomplishment . . .
. . . of loneliness . . .
The muscular feeling of swimming through water . . .
. . . of running through a park . . .
. . . of rowing a boat . . .

Allow yourself just to relax another few moments and then feel yourself come back to an awareness of where you really are.

Practicing these exercises over and over will help you use visualization as a practical tool in your nutrition program, in your exercise program and in your pursuit of excellence in your everyday life.

THE POWER OF SELF-TALK

When your mind talks, your body listens! Research has shown that our thoughts can raise and lower body temperature, secrete hormones, relax muscles and nerve endings, dilate and constrict arteries and raise and lower pulse rate. With this evidence it is obvious that we need to control the language we use on ourselves.

Winners rarely put themselves down in words before or after a performance; they use positive feedforward self-talk and positive feedback self-talk as part of their training programs until it becomes a force of habit. They say "I can. . . . I will. . . . Next time I'll get it right. . . . I'm feeling better. . . . I'm ready. . . . Thank you." Losers fall into the trap of saying: "I can't. . . . "I'm a klutz. . . . I can't stay in shape. . . . I wish . . . If only . . . "I shoulda . . . "Yeah, but . . ."

You are your most important critic. There is no opinion as vitally important to your fitness and well-being as the opinion you have of yourself. The most important meetings, briefings, coaching sessions and conversations you'll ever have are the conversations you will have with yourself.

As you read this you're talking to yourself: "Let's see if I understand what they mean by that. . . . How does that compare with my own experiences. . . . I already knew that. . . . I think I'll try that."

We believe that this self-talk is critical in Quantum Fitness and can be controlled to work for us in achieving our Quantum goals of health, performance and longevity. In our previous research with astronauts, executives and other individuals functioning under pressure, and in our continuing observation of Olympic athletes throughout the world, there is a technique of "scripting" self-talk that seems to be the most effective; it is known as affirmation. The Olympic athletes call this technique self-statement; the astronauts call it simulation. In the Quantum Fitness program we use feedforward (preplay) and feedback (replay) statements. When you apply feedforward techniques to your daily perform-ance, and review that performance with feedback techniques, you have the second major Quantum access code, the simulation cycle.

THE SIMULATION CYCLE IN QUANTUM FITNESS

To simulate means to act like or look like something. In order for you to get ready for the Quantum leap in fitness, you must under-stand that a simulation is a preview of coming attractions, *not* wishful thinking. If you ever doubt the value of simulation and self-talk, just think back to when the astronauts were preparing for the *Apollo* moon program. How would you feel if some theoretical scientists said they were going to sit you on top of a Titan missile and send you a half-million miles in orbital flight, land you on the moon and bring you home using experimental equipment that had been built by the lowest bidder?

The *Apollo* astronauts were masters of simulation. They prac-ticed bobbing up and down in rubber rafts at sea and they floated in simulation chambers subjected to negative gravity forces, re-sponding to the feeling of weightlessness to be experienced in outer space. They practiced on desert terrain with a simulated lunar excursion module as if they were landing it on the surface of the moon. Hour after hour, month after month, they memorized and simulated the hundreds of steps that made up the vital se-quences that NASA officials had imagined and computed would take them safely to the moon and back.

When Neil Armstrong landed the *Eagle* on the lunar surface, he said, "It was beautiful, just like our drills." On a later moon expe-dition *Apollo* Captain Charles Conrad, junior, commented, "It's just like old-home week. I feel like I've been here many times be-fore. After all, we've been rehearsing this moment for the past four years!"

We are astronauts too! The Quantum program is taking us on a voyage into inner space where we are discovering that fitness is as much a state of mind as it is a condition of our body. We are the scriptwriters, the directors and the stars of either an Oscar-winning epic or a Grade-B movie. We can devastate or elevate our previews of coming attractions. We can be sarcastic or enthusiastic in our reviews of our daily performances. Your self-talk is being monitored and recorded, minute to minute, by your self-image. And your self-image is formed as a result of verbal, visual and emotional thought patterns within your mind, which you can learn to control.

There are three basic types of simulation feedforward and feedback self-statements:

(1) *General self-talk.* These are affirmative statements that can be used at any time and place for a feeling of general well-being. Examples:

"I like myself."
"I'm glad I'm me."
"I'm relaxing now. I am at peace."
"I'm in control of my body."
"I feel that my body is more healthy now."
"I give the best of me in everything."
"I am strong and full of energy."
"I respect and appreciate myself."
"I'm a winner."

(2) *Specific self-talk.* These statements are used to project and reaffirm our specific skills, goals and attributes. Examples:

"I weight 115 pounds and feel trim in my bathing suit."
"I drink a glass of water with every meal."
"My food contains enough salt naturally; I don't need to add any."
"I eat fish or poultry to get my lean protein."

44

"I eat small portions of nourishing food at regular intervals."

"My stomach is flat."

"My pulse rate is sixty beats per minute while resting."

"My back muscles are relaxed and flexible."

"I enjoy bike-riding on the weekend."

"I listen to my body talk and know the limits of my endurance."

"My breathing is relaxed and effortless."

"I am taking the quantum leap because my mind, nutrition program and exercise program are in harmony."

(3) *Process self-talk.* These are one- or two-word self-statements that can be used as "trigger" ideas at mealtime, during an exercise workout or during the performance of professional, sporting or other demanding skills. Examples:

"Concentrate."

"Focus."

"Backhand follow-through."

"Easy."

"Push-off."

"Explode now."

"Relax."

"Power on."

"Think thin."

"Smooth."

"Strong."

"Vital."

"Healthy."

In order for these simulation self-statements to be most effective it is extremely important to construct and phrase them properly. Here are specific guidelines for you to use in developing a simulation cycle that will strengthen your eating habits, your exercise habits, your mental habits and your professional and personal lifestyle.

(1) Make the decision to turn negative self-talk into positive

45

self-talk. Listen to what you are saying and thinking in anticipation of and in response to your daily challenges. Become aware of your own negative self-talk and construct affirmative self-talk statements in their place.

(2) Respond rather than react to the negative self-talk of others. Learn to recall your adaptive relaxation and autogenic exercise training. The next time someone offers you some of his or her negative statements, don't agree mentally. You can learn either to ignore the comment and say nothing, or turn it around and help that person with your positive response to the comment.

(3) Direct your self-talk *toward what you desire* instead of trying to come away from what you don't want. Your mind can't concentrate on the reverse of an idea. If you try to tell yourself not to repeat mistakes, your mind will reinforce the mistake. You want to focus your current dominant thought on your desires, not your dislikes. *This is critically important.*

Effective: "I am in control of my habits."
"I weigh a slim, trim 125 pounds."
"I arrive early for appointments."
"I am patient and loving with my children."

Ineffective: "I can quit smoking."
"I'm too fat and have to lose weight."
"I won't be late anymore."
"I won't yell at the children."

(4) Always use personal pronouns. Words such as *I, my* and *me* will personalize your statements and make them easier to internalize.

Effective: "I enjoy jogging three times a week."
Ineffective: "Jogging is good exercise."

(5) Keep your self-talk in the present tense. Referring to the past or future may be counterproductive to making progress.

Effective: "I enjoy good health and physical fitness."
Ineffective: "Someday I'll get in good physical condition."

(6) Keep your self-talk noncompetitive instead of measuring yourself against others.

Effective: "I am starting on the team and doing the job well."

Ineffective: "I will beat John out of the starting position."

(7) In writing your statements, concentrate on incremental improvement over your previous measured performance. Don't strive for perfection or unrealistic superhuman efforts.

Effective: "I clear the bar at six feet, a new record for me."

Ineffective: "I'm the best in the world in the high jump."

Once you have correctly constructed simulation statements for your Quantum goals, write these statements on cards or in a notebook, or record them in your own voice on an audio cassette tape. Read or listen to the statements at the beginning of your normal routine, get to know them during the day and review them again before you retire at night. Visualize yourself as having already reached each goal you are simulating. Allow yourself actually to feel the pride of doing well. Don't let the technique of simulation give you the false impression that you are brainwashing or kidding yourself. On the contrary, we are suggesting just the opposite. We are unconsciously being brainwashed by the television shows and movies we watch, by the magazines we read and by the people we talk to; all of these are giving us a sensationalized perception of what is happening in the world. Much of what we see and hear is negative, because bad news attracts more attention and sells better. Isn't it time we concentrated on information designed for our success rather than our distress? Brainwashing is what happens when you get hooked on television. Quantum Fitness is what happens when you get hooked on your simulated goals.

By combining the techniques of adaptive relaxation, visualization and self-talk, you will set in motion the Quantum simulation cycle. Your feedforward self-talk will preplay a positive self-image about specific activities in your fitness profile. Your performance will improve because of your elevated self-image, and sometimes your performance will exceed your expectations. Your feedback self-talk will say "Good for me, now we're getting somewhere." On occasion your performance will fall short of your expectations. Your feedback self-talk will say "Next time we'll do better. Let's make a target correction to help get it right." One of the secrets of the Quantum mind is that our responses to our performances—in words, images and feelings—are just as important as our self-images or simulations of ourselves before we ever attempt to perform in the first place.

THE MIRROR IN YOUR MIND

When you look in the mirror, you see two reflections. You see the person you are today and the person you will become. Step back from your life today and take a long walk, bike ride or jog on the beach, or in the woods, or by a lake, or up a mountain trail. Observe the wonder of and abundance in nature, and remember that everything in your world and your body is totally interconnected. Listen to the subtle rhythms in your outer and inner environment. Recognize that while there are constant rhythms around you and within you, that there is also the rhythm of change to which you must constantly adapt.

As you relax and open up, make an honest assessment of what you are doing, where you are going in your life and who you are becoming. Understand the marvel of your own uniqueness and remember the Quantum principle that you cause everything to be different by your involvement and your actions. Realize how you have been selling yourself short in evaluating your own potential. By looking at the "impossible" in a different way, suddenly you see the never-ending possibilities.

Your true potential is in the mirror of your mind. It is your source for tomorrow's dreams and it is the force for today's decisions. Isn't it time you stepped through the looking glass? Let's take the next step together.

QUANTUM NUTRITION

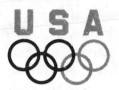

BIOFIRES—the tiny energy suns that power our cells, our organs, our muscles and our minds—burn in Olympic athletes just as they burn in you

Imagine yourself in the Olympic Village of the Olympic Games. It is a city unlike any other on earth, housing thousands of elite athletes from more countries than sit at the United Nations. But how can all those athletes be fed? How can the tastes, habits and diets of athletes from more than 150 countries be satisfied? Paradoxically the answer lies in a question: How is it that all these athletes eat differently—sometimes *very* differently—yet, all drive their bodies toward the limits of human athletic performance? Why is it that dinner as varied as stir-fried bean curd with vegetables, or Indonesian *rijstaffel*, or Armenian *harpoot kufta* (lamb and cracked wheat balls filled with currants and pine nuts) can all power that athlete sitting across from you to a gold-medal performance? Our answer: The biofires within us all burn on the same basic fuels. Those Olympic Village chefs are going to prepare a great variety of dishes and satisfy a great number of palates, but they are going to fuel all those biofires by careful and intelligent inclusion of the basic nutrients.

Olympic champions have access to no miracle foods and follow no miracle diets. They, like you, must draw upon a balanced variety of foods, providing nutrients in a variety of combinations. They, like you, must discern fact from fancy in the complex maze of foods and diet strategies.

We're going to prepare you for a *nutritional* Quantum leap, past the seemingly endless discoveries about physiology, metabolism and weight control. Our first step is the application of the Quantum Force. Much more than "you are what you eat," you are what you *think*.

THE QUANTUM FORCE: YOU ARE WHAT YOU THINK

Think of your mind as your *most important digestive organ.*

If you put "junk food" into your mind, you will be malnourished. If you put a variety of positive, balanced thoughts into your mind, you will get a healthier body as a result. How is it that Americans have been dieting steadily for nearly thirty years and have gained about ten pounds per person in the process? Why are we more bulimic, anorexic, fad-diet fanatical and frenetic about food than ever before? Where did we go wrong?

In our opinion the culprit is a familiar two-word phrase: *instant gratification.* If it feels good right away, we'll try it. If we can lose ten pounds by that vacation, we'll do it. If it may mean cancer in thirty years, why, that's thirty years away! For many Americans the attitude has become "I want the American dream I saw on TV, and I want it now. Make me slim, good-looking and healthy. Give me something I can swallow, quick!"

Eating is and always has been the great pacifier, the prime sub-stitute for real success. From infancy on, we have been trained to stuff something in our mouths to overcome frustration. Even in today's nutrition-conscious society, mothers placate their tan-trum-throwers and whiners with granola bars instead of the Oreos and ginger snaps of an earlier generation.

But we can't have it both ways. If we want positive results, we must pay the price, and the price for good nutrition is a persever-ing mind-set that is practiced every day, just like brushing our teeth. The fad-diet syndrome is a vicious negative cycle that is doomed to failure. Each new diet program we try—even if it "works wonders" for a while—reinforces our past experiences of failure. By the very act of going *on* a diet, it is a foregone conclu-sion that at some point we will be going *off* the same diet. When we are on a diet, we feel noble but deprived. When we go off the diet, we feel relieved but terribly guilty. The guilt keeps our self-image low, and our performance level plunges to meet the low self-image.

Obesity and poor nutrition are "habit disorders," which means that they are, in part, caused by behavior patterns that must be changed. The all-important connections between the mind, nutri-tion and life-style have gone awry. You *can* turn disorder into order, though, by applying the Quantum mental access codes to the Quantum Nutrition access codes and then adding the missing link of Quantum Exercise as the finishing touch.

Make the Quantum principles your food for thought by using the exercises at the end of this chapter. Select those self-talk simu-lations that will put the Quantum nutrition principles into your daily routine. As you begin applying the Quantum Force program from Chapter Two to your eating habits, you will learn to develop your own simulations, fine-tuning them to meet your specific needs.

The Primary Principle: Variety

As a person concerned about nutrition, you know by now that there are no magic foods or miracle diets. The key to proper nutrition is *variety*. Selecting from the widest possible variety of good foods is your single most important nutritional strategy. There is simply no better way to maximize the chances of getting all required nutrients and minimize the risks of ingesting too many toxic substances. Many Americans unconsciously limit their food choices to as few as ten or fifteen items, always depending on that small number for complete nourishment. The chances are staggeringly low that their complete nutrient needs can be met by so few foods.

Conversely, should you have an adverse reaction to particular food substances (a common phenomenon), or should your typical food choices contain even small amounts of carcinogens or other dangerous compounds, repeated exposure could be quite hazardous.

You have several well-developed defense mechanisms against poisons. Your front line of defense is taste: Food and other substances that are toxic usually taste wrong. If this defense is overcome, your digestive organs may refuse the food in either of two directions: up and out (by vomiting) or down and out (diarrhea). Finally, your liver serves as a detoxification plant, filtering and altering substances that it knows to be hazardous. Alcohol, for example, in small enough amounts, can be broken down by a special liver enzyme and excreted through the urine.

If you lived your life as a laboratory experiment, strapped to a stainless-steel table, with machines intravenously supplying specific portions of nutrients as your body needed them, you would have a chance to achieve the ideal balanced diet (within the bounds of present knowledge). Although none of us would want to be the subject of such an experiment, you may feel that your present diet is only a few steps removed from that kind of scientific torture. Being "strapped" to a particular diet, constantly counting calories and/or carbohydrates, can be as boring and tedious as our laboratory scene.

Fortunately we do not have to suffer under such rigid requirements. A trip to the grocery store can enable you to enjoy the richest supply of foodstuffs in the world, foods that are not only good for you but good to eat. By eating an intelligent variety of good foods, the probability of ingesting proper nutrients for your body is increased. The access codes to come will supply you with information on what foods are *good* foods; however, the joy of selecting from America's cornucopia is strictly up to you!

Rhythms, Large and Small

They are there, in systems as small as your cells and as large as the universe. Some can be seen, felt or sensed, and some defy close experimental scrutiny. Chronobiology, the science that studies the rhythms of living systems, is the newest and most promising direction of our Olympic research program. A team of NASA chronobiologists, headquartered at Harvard University, is outlining how our Olympic athletes can best listen to their rhythms and make use of them. It will work for you as well.

The most practical outcome of recent rhythm research is the discovery that humans function most efficiently on smaller and more frequent meals than the traditional breakfast, lunch, and dinner. There are a number of beneficial effects when you break your daily intake of calories into four equally caloric meals: The smaller quantities of foods are easier to digest; blood sugar and insulin levels remain more stable; and hunger is moderated more efficiently. Your energy level stays high and constant, and most important, food is metabolized, or used more quickly after each meal and is not shunted along the metabolic pathway to fat storage.

Think of a bathtub with a one-inch drain. Add water at a slow enough rate and the tub will never overflow. Add water too quickly and you'll slosh around in the results. Your body works on very much the same principle. Four equally caloric meals will flow smoothly down the metabolic pipeline. Large meals will overflow—and the body stores overflow calories as fat.

Adaptation: Use and Abuse

The human being's marvelous and limitless ability to adapt is more often its downfall than its salvation. Our bodies will adapt, or sometimes *maladapt*, to any conditions we offer it. If you are overweight or unfit, you have adapted to poor nutrition and poor exercise quite well, and the results of that *mal*adaptation are seen in less-than-optimal health, sub-par performance and reduced longevity.

Unfortunately, you can't appreciate your condition without knowing how the Quantum you can feel. You're not *really* sick, so you don't have a feel for what optimal health may be. You make it through each day, and usually squeeze in a few hours of good sleep, but you can't appreciate a lust for activity, doing, being. And you can't see your longevity being compromised each day.

But the Quantum you can know about health, performance and longevity. You can construct your life so that you think right, eat right and exercise right. You can adapt to a varied, high-energy, successful life, not to a slower metabolism from a day of inactivity. Not to the same six foods. Not to irregular attempts to jog your way to the nadir of fitness.

Stay with us: You *can* begin the readaptation process quite easily. Follow us from the mind to the functioning body and the dynamics of metabolism and weight control.

WEIGHT-CONTROL DYNAMICS

Dieting doesn't work. We know that all biofires burn by the same physical laws, and that energy put into a system must always be balanced by energy out. Yet, mysteriously, the balance struck between food calories in and exercise calories out rarely results in the expected weight change. The thin seem to remain thin, despite their efforts to gain weight, and the overweight remain overweight, despite efforts to slim down.

Hardly. Recent trends in obesity research point out that the body's weight-control system is far more complicated than was ever imagined. Weight control requires a Quantum attack: mind, nutrition and exercise. No single diet, exercise strategy or mind-set can alter the unhealthy balance you've settled at. But the only safe, effective and long-term method of weight control is still the one dictated by the laws of thermodynamics: If, over the long-haul, energy expenditure exceeds energy intake, you will lose body weight.

The Body Knows

Researchers are now in general agreement that the body somehow senses both the storage of fat and efforts to increase or decrease the amount of fat stored. Several fascinating studies have demonstrated that appetite, eating behaviors and even mental/emotional function may vary, based on changes in the amount of body fat. One study, almost frightening in its evidence of "body intelligence," took place at the University of Pennsylvania laboratory of psychiatrist Henry Jordan. Colleague Theresa Spiegel slowly adapted her volunteer group to a diet consisting of a milk-shakelike diet drink. Over the course of several days her subjects came to obtain their sum total of daily calories (about 3,000) from a stainless-steel nipple connected to reservoirs of flavored liquid. Without informing her volunteers, Spiegel then cut the caloric concentration of the mix in half. The solution was adjusted for taste and texture, and in fact few of the subjects noticed the change. The amounts of liquid consumed rose inexorably. Within the space of several days the subjects were drinking twice as much of the drink and obtaining the same number of calories as before the dilution was performed. Obviously some physiological feed-

55

back mechanism sensed the reduction in calories and was able to effect a subconscious change in eating behavior to compensate.

The Set-Point Theory

There is now significant evidence that your body has armed itself with set-point, a level of body fatness that is physiologically "comfortable." It has not chosen this equilibrium level arbitrarily, however; it is a function of many variables, some of which can be altered.

Proponents of the set-point theory hold that your metabolic rate speeds or slows to keep you at your fat equilibrium. Reduce your daily caloric intake to lose body fat and your metabolism not-so-obligingly slows down. Though you're eating less, you're also burning less. The net result: no change.

Increase your caloric intake slightly and you find that metabolism speeds up. Through a mechanism that may include a type of excess-calorie–burning tissue called "brown fat," you burn more while eating more. Overpower this calorie-overflow system and you risk creeping obesity. Higher calorie intakes, coupled with gradually decreasing activity levels, may add several pounds a year as you age.

Can this somewhat hypothetical set-point be changed? It appears so, although there is still more work to be done. Your most effective weapon appears to be exercise. Sustained increases in physical activity seem to raise your metabolism and lower your level of body fat.

Lest you get the wrong message here, the possible existence of a stubborn set-point relieves you of *none* of the responsibility for the optimal selection of foods. You can still choose the foods that will optimize health, performance and longevity. And you can still structure your food choices and meals so that hunger is tamed and digestion is most efficient.

Beating the Wrong Equilibrium Setting

Science and technology offer us several types of assistance in breaking away from a maladapted state. We've mentioned two major strategies already: Eating a larger number of smaller meals decreases the probability that calories in excess of immediate post-meal needs will be stored as fat; and exercise seems to be the key tool in lowering a possible set-point for body fat.

Insulin response is the weighty-sounding phenomenon being studied in several arenas today. Leading researcher Judith Rodin, Ph.D., of Yale University, has demonstrated that foods differ in their effect on hunger-causing insulin production. Debunking the myth that blood sugar alone carries the hunger message, Rodin and her colleagues have shown in several studies how powerful the effects of insulin may be. Subjects in the Rodin studies who consumed foods that minimally effect insulin production ate less and were less hungry than those who ate insulin-stimulating foods.

What are the choices particularly effective in satisfying your hunger without boosting blood sugar and insulin production? Fructose, whole-wheat and white pasta, apples, oranges, sweet potatoes, skim milk, peas and beans. Surprised? Whole wheat bread causes a rise in blood sugar twice as fast as ice cream. White baking potatoes cause a faster rise in blood sugar than a candy bar. Of course, this does *not* mean that you should rush out for foods that are easy on your blood sugar but often nutritionally incomplete. And what's more, other researchers caution that these numbers were calculated when foods were consumed in isolation. As part of an entire meal, the items noted above may cause quite different blood-sugar responses. In any case, Rodin and her colleagues are busy at further detailing the food-insulin-glucose-appetite interplay.

Another important scientific contribution to your battle against a maladapted state is body composition assessment. Body composition analysis is rightfully making Americans *fat*-conscious instead of *weight*-conscious. It's not what you *weigh* that counts; it's the proportion of fat and lean tissue. Through any of several techniques, the amounts of lean (muscle, bone, organ) and fat tissue in your body can be determined.

Your old bathroom scale can report only gross changes in weight; it can't distinguish fat loss from muscle atrophy, or fat gain from muscle gain. An unbalanced diet will cause a weight loss that is an astounding 50 percent lean tissue (water and muscle) and 50 percent fat, *not* the 100 percent fat the ads will lead you to expect. Use your scale and be lulled into a false sense of dietary and muscular security. Then there's the frequent case where the individual exercises while dieting (losing fat while adding muscle) and quits upon reuse of the bathroom scale and the discovery that his or her body weight is unchanged.

Since advanced techniques such as ultrasound, electrical conductivity and hydrostatic (underwater) weighing are beyond home use, how can you determine your body composition on your own? The "pinch an inch" test, where you grab a pinch-full of skin and fat, is a step in the right direction. Up until recently it was the only at-home approximation of the "skinfold technique," where measured pinches of skin and fat from specific sites around the body are used to predict accurately the fat percentage of your body weight. Technology has come through again, though, and a reliable, accurate and surprisingly inexpensive skinfold device now exists for home use.*

We strongly advise that you take advantage of body-composition assessment technologies. Whether it's at a fitness center, at a medical checkup or at home, the knowledge you gain will add immeasurably to your quest for the Quantum goals.

* The Fat-O-Meter is available from Omni Fitness Services, 355-8F South End Avenue, New York, NY, 10280 for $9.95 plus $2.00 for shipping and handling.

YOU CAN FOOL ALL OF THE PEOPLE . . . OR, FOOD MYTHS AND TRUTHS

Someone once said that old myths die hard. We're afraid that some of these nutritional old-wives' rules will *never* die! We would like nothing more than to have you take a Quantum leap across these next several pages right now. Unfortunately, the probability is quite high that you'll be surprised at how much you never knew or thought you knew but didn't.

Let's clear the air and then proceed with your Quantum access codes.

Carbohydrates

MYTH: "Carbohydrates are bad for you."

TRUTH: No fuel source is "bad" for you in and of itself unless taken in excess. The *right* carbohydrates, such as cereals, fruits and vegetables, are critically important nutrient sources for your mind and body, and optimally make up 60 to 70 percent of your daily caloric intake. Carbohydrates are the most efficiently-burnable fuels, and frequently include other biologically valuable compounds—fiber and fructose, for example. To be consumed in moderation: carbohydrates that occur as refined sugar.

MYTH: "Low-carbohydrate diets are the most effective because they force the body to burn fat as fuel."

TRUTH: This runs a close second in the contest to see which myth has fooled more people. Your body is torn from an equilibrium state when it is deprived of carbohydrates. Since complete fat breakdown can occur only if carbohydrates are present, incomplete fat breakdown products, called ketone bodies, course through your circulatory system. These ketone bodies produce a host of deleterious results, including nausea, fatigue, apathy and possible brain damage. Perhaps the most obvious sign of ketosis is the telltale odor of acetone on the breath of a low-carbohydrate dieter.

59

What's more, faced with a cutoff of its major fuel supply, the body turns quickly and easily to a third fuel source: protein. Protein burned for energy cannot be used for growth and maintenance of body tissue, and it is quite common for 50 percent of the weight loss from a low-carbohydrate diet to come from muscle and water. The goal of a diet is to lose fat, not muscle.

Proteins

MYTH: "Protein is the most important energy source in fitness and athletic conditioning; therefore, steak is a must for every training table."

TRUTH: The body's main priority is the requirement for energy. Protein functions as an energy source only when insufficient fat and carbohydrates are eaten. (By the way, steaks are 30 to 50 percent fat!)

MYTH: "You can never eat too much protein."

TRUTH: The consumption of more than your daily requirement of protein stresses your entire metabolic system. Abnormal enlargement of the liver and kidneys has been noted in cases of extremely high protein intake.

MYTH: "Athletes in training cannot meet their protein needs through normal dietary means."

TRUTH: Athletic training, pregnancy and adolescent growth all raise protein needs, but these elevated needs can still be easily met through a proper selection of protein foods. No reputable scientist has ever produced a scrap of evidence that protein supplements are necessary or effective.

Fats

MYTH: "All dietary fat should be carefully avoided."

TRUTH: While it is true that many scientists believe that Americans consume too much dietary fat, at least 20 percent of your daily caloric intake should come from that source (we're now in the 40-to-50-percent range). Several components of dietary fat, primarily the essential fatty acids, are essential to normal, healthy functioning.

In addition to being a major source of energy, fats are important constituents of all cells in the body. They help transport fat-soluble nutrients, namely vitamins A, D, E and K, maintain body temperature, add desirable flavor to foods and help satisfy hunger.

MYTH: "Cholesterol in foods is the primary cause of heart attacks, strokes and other vascular disorders."

TRUTH: Cholesterol is *one* of several significant factors that contribute to these conditions. Since the level of cholesterol in your blood is affected by the amount of saturated fat you consume, the percentage of saturated fat in your diet should be reduced.

Since fats are often found in combination with animal protein, you should stress fish, skinless poultry and lean cuts of meat, along with a variety of fat-free plant protein sources, in your diet. If cooking requires shortening or oil, the polyunsaturated oils are best.

Finally, as we'll see later, there are three major types of cholesterol, one of which may actually help remove deposits of fatty plaque from arterial walls.

Fiber

MYTH: "The only way to obtain sufficient dietary fiber is to use bran-type supplements."

TRUTH: A varied selection of good foods, such as vegetables, fruits and cereals, more than satisfies your daily fiber needs.

Fluids

MYTH: "Commercially prepared sport drinks [electrolyte solutions] replace bodily fluids more quickly than other liquids."

TRUTH: Scientists have swung back to clear, cold water as the ultimate fluid-replacement beverage. Most commercial drinks are actually absorbed more slowly than water, and there is no strong evidence that we lose enough electrolytes (minerals in bodily fluids) during most forms of exercise to require their immediate replacement.

MYTH: "Since fluids are so important to my well-being, I can take them in any form—coffee, tea, soft drinks, etc."

TRUTH: Only clear water contains no caffeine, no coloring, no additives and no refined sugar. Occasional intake of other fluids is certainly fine, but water is the number-one choice.

MYTH: "Cold beverages are dangerous when exercising in the heat."

TRUTH: The opposite is actually the case: Cold fluids are absorbed far more rapidly than warmer ones, and therefore reduce the chances of heat disorders from dehydration.

Vitamins and Minerals

MYTH: "My diet can't provide all the necessary vitamins and minerals."

TRUTH: Given a varied and intelligent selection of foods, preparations and cooking methods, this is hogwash. Your diet can certainly provide all necessary nutrients. Women should take extra care in obtaining calcium and iron, the two minerals they are most frequently deficient in. Additional supplementation is not necessary if enough natural-source minerals can be obtained. Pregnant and nursing women should consult their doctors for specific nutritional guidelines.

MYTH: "Fruits and vegetables grown in nutrient-depleted soil will themselves be depleted of essential nutrients."

TRUTH: This one is a favorite of your local organic grocer, but it's not true.

Natural Foods

MYTH: "Natural foods are better."

TRUTH: We would easily fill a book debunking this myth. Yes, modern food-processing does result in diminished nutrient levels in some cases, but often some of these nutrients are replaced. And as a matter of fact, the *lack* of adequate processing may increase the risk of botulism and salmonellosis. While we are not sure that all food additives are safe, natural foods may contain all sorts of natural poisons. The natural peanut butter you buy at your health food store contains high levels of aflotoxin, a direct cause of liver cancer. No scientifically creditable study has ever shown "natural" or "organic" foods (whatever they may be) to be superior to meats, dairy products, produce and processed foods that you can buy in the supermarket. It's up to you to decide if the health risks and higher prices are worth it.

Vegetables

MYTH: "Fresh vegetables are always better than frozen."

TRUTH: If you buy from a local farmstand, yes. If your vegetables are picked in Washington State, stored a day, trucked to New York and allowed to sit on the shelf for three days, you may be better off with frozen. Look for those frozen vegetables that are processed on the day they are picked; several food packers are now prominently advertising the fact on their labels.

MYTH: "Raw vegetables are always better than cooked vegetables."

TRUTH: This is true if you soak your vegetables for long periods of time, or boil them until they are limp and mushy. However, steaming breaks down starch granules and makes vegetables more easily digestible, without decreasing nutritive content.

Miracle Foods

MYTH: "There are foods, such as spirulina, bee pollen and yogurt, that will work miracles."

TRUTH: There are no foods that work miracles.

Weight Control

MYTH: "Eating fewer meals will help me lose weight."

TRUTH: The opposite is true. As we've noted above, research

has clearly shown the weight-control benefits of smaller and *more frequent* meals.

MYTH: "Fat people eat too much."

TRUTH: Again, the opposite is true. Fat people have mal-adapted to their reduced activity level, and frequently eat less than their lean counterparts.

MYTH: "I must count calories to lose weight."

TRUTH: The caloric values of the foods you eat and the activities you perform vary too widely to make calorie-counting effective. Balanced variety in food selection and exercise are the keys to weight control.

MYTH: "Snacking between meals makes you fat."

TRUTH: Here's some good news: Intelligent between-meal snacks can effectively stabilize hunger, add nutritional benefit and make adherence to a dietary regimen easier. Fruits and vegetables are top choices for snacks.

MYTH: Nuts and dried fruits are excellent health foods for weight control.

TRUTH: Both nuts and dried fruits are calorie-dense, even though they contain fiber. Because dried fruits such as apricots, raisins, pears, figs and dates have most of their water removed, they are a highly concentrated source of sugar. Nuts, on the other hand, contain substantial amounts of fat. Because both nuts and dried fruit are easy to nibble on continuously, the weight-conscious person should eat them with discretion.

MYTH: "I inherited a fat body."

TRUTH: There are some people who do have metabolic problems, however, most people are overweight because of their eating and exercise habits. People with normal metabolisms burn calories in direct relation to the calories they expend, but regardless of your inheritance, you can recondition your mind to learn new habits that will help compensate for your genes.

MYTH: "Exercise doesn't burn enough calories to make a difference."

TRUTH: The confirmed exercise-hater revels in the thought that it takes about twelve hours of walking to burn one pound of fat. However, the value of exercise in weight control, even in small doses, could not be clearer. Regular exercise elevates metabolism both in the short run (for hours after you exercise) and in the long run (by creating permanent changes in the basal metabolic rate). The result is that more calories are continually being burned, even when you are at rest.

MYTH: "You can spot-reduce any area of the body through intense and focused exercise."

TRUTH: While the muscles underlying a cosmetically bothersome region like your abdomen or thighs may tone or grow with exercise, fat will *not* be preferentially burned from those areas. The body breaks down fat from genetically programmed areas, *not* where you exercise.

MYTH: Plastic suits, belts and wraps are wonderfully easy ways to melt fat away."

TRUTH: We're glad you have a sense of humor. They're all worthless.

The Mind

MYTH: "Fat people are happier."

TRUTH: *Fit* people are happier. Many fat people feel rejected and embarrassed. Many underweight people also worry about their appearance. People who accept themselves as imperfect, but changing and improving, are the happiest. Also, individuals who are physically fit are more optimistic. They may produce more morphinelike substances, called endorphins, in their brains; these give them a "natural high."

MYTH: "I eat like a bird but still gain weight."

TRUTH: If you ate like a bird, you would consume more than two times your own weight in food every day. Birds eat almost all day long. The best thing about birds' diet habits is that most of them concentrate on whole-grain or fiber-rich food.

MYTH: "Fat people are neurotic."

TRUTH: Given the famous Rorschach test, groups of fat people cannot be reliably distinguished from groups of normal-weight individuals. Overweight people, however, do tend to use eating to compensate for depression and anxiety. Fit people use adaptive relaxation and physical exercise to counter depression and anxiety.

MYTH: "I can't control my eating habits."

TRUTH: You can control your eating, smoking, sleeping, work, nail-biting, dental hygiene and exercise habits. Behavior is learned. By using adaptive relaxation techniques to put the mind in a receptive state, visualization and simulation self-talk exercises can be rehearsed to foster new, positive habits. Habits begin as offhanded notions, then with repetition become unbreakable cables to shackle or strengthen our lives.

NUTRITION IN PROPER CONTEXT: THE QUANTUM ACCESS CODES

Knowledge without context is worthless. Knowing what each of an automobile's two thousand parts does will leave you waiting without transportation unless you understand their context: how they fit together.

Thousands of nutritional choices lay spread out before you: the diets, the miracle foods, the supplements, the advice of the National Livestock and Meat Board, and the National Dairy Council and the many government agencies and the food companies. You don't need to be reminded that there's simply no context in which to order the information. Or at least there wasn't before Quantum Fitness.

By applying the Quantum access codes of fiber-based carbohydrates, lean source protein and clear water to the Quantum principles of variety, adaptability and rhythm, you will make simple, logical sense out of the nutritional universe.

Fiber-Based Carbohydrates: Fuel for the Biofires

We find it more than interesting that natural, unrefined carbohydrates—the kind found in whole grains, vegetables, beans and fruits—is the only nutrient category *not* linked to any debilitating or deadly diseases. Since the ultimate test of a carbohydrate's value to you is the presence or absence of fiber—generally foods containing naturally occurring carbohydrates have it; most refined ones don't—we call access code number one fiber-based carbohydrates. As sources of your body's primary energy fuel and the *only* sources of the all-important non-digestible compound called fiber, these naturally occurring carbohydrates (which are often laden with protein and contain no fat) will be your major dietary staple.

Carbohydrates occur in two basic forms: starches, which are called *complex* carbohydrates, and sugars, called *simple* carbohydrates. "Natural" carbohydrates may be simple or complex and are found in unprocessed foods from the earth.

Natural carbohydrates are also nutrient-dense and give you more bang for your caloric buck. How's this for nutritional value? One five ounce, 110-calorie white potato provides significant percentages of protein, iron, phosphorous, thiamine, niacin, vitamins C and B_6, copper, magnesium, iodine and folic acid.

Refined carbohydrates, like white sugar, are produced from the original, natural sources, and are usually added to foods that don't otherwise contain them. The many foods that contain added, refined carbohydrates often contain a low percentage of nutrients but are high in calories. For example, three plain sugar cookies contain the same number of calories as the previously mentioned potato, but almost none of the nutrient value.

As we mentioned earlier, foods high in natural carbohydrates are the primary sources of dietary fiber. Fiber supplies neither calories nor nutrients; it provides roughage for the digestive system. Links, some of them fairly substantial, have been established over the past ten years between increases in dietary fiber and:

- improvement of bowel regularity (fiber absorbs water in the colon, which softens stool)
- lower, incidence of hemorrhoids, diverticulosis and spastic colon by improving regularity
- reduction in diabetic symptoms and the need for insulin
- reduction of the risk of coronary artery disease
- improved weight control.

Fiber-containing foods are nutrient-dense, filling and low in calories. But don't swallow that bottle of bran just yet. All dietary fiber is not created equal. Bran, the most widely known source of fiber, is more than 90 percent cellulose, a compound that forms the cell walls of plants. Bran intake has been noted to have either an insubstantial or possibly negative effect on blood cholesterol levels. On the other hand, water-soluble fiber sources such as pectins (fruits), guar gum (beans) carrots and rolled oats can significantly lower blood cholesterol and triglycerides. (The effect may result from these fibers' ability to increase the elimination of bile acids, which are made from cholesterol.) As we've said again and again, variety is the key to nutritional optimization. By selecting from a wide spectrum of fiber-based carbohydrates, you can maximize the chances of obtaining all the sources of fiber you need.

Variety also reduces the chances of toxic effects from overconsumption of one fiber source. Whole wheat and other whole grains, while nutrient-dense and fiber-rich, also contain a compound called phytic acid, which can combine with calcium, iron and zinc and prevent the body from absorbing these minerals properly.

A second effect of large, sudden increases in fiber consumption is intestinal gas formation during fiber digestion. The bacteria in the large intestine act upon fiber, and such gases as carbon dioxide, hydrogen and methane can be produced. Problems with intestinal gas can be minimized through slow increases in dietary fiber consumption. In most Americans the adjustment to an increase in fiber can occur within a matter of weeks, but the elderly, the poorly nourished and adolescents are advised to avoid radical increases in dietary fiber.

We've incorporated what's known about fiber-based carbohydrates into our selection tables below. Remember that raw fruits and vegetables, whole grains and legumes (dried peas and beans) are your top choices. And don't forget variety!

VEGETABLES, LEGUMES, SPROUTS

Alfalfa
Artichokes
Asparagus
Bamboo shoots
Beet greens
Beets
Broccoli
Brussels sprouts
Cabbage (Chinese, common, red, savoy)
Carrots
Cauliflower
Celeriac root
Celery
Chard
Chives
Collard greens
Corn
Cress (sprigs)
Cucumbers
Dandelion greens
Dock (sorrel)
Eggplant
Endives

Garlic
Ginger root
Jerusalem artichokes
Kale
Kohlrabi
Leeks
Legumes (all beans, including azuki, black, black-eyed peas, chick-peas [garbanzos], green, kidney, lentils, lentil sprouts, lima, mung sprouts, peanuts, pinto, soybeans, soybean curd [tofu], snap, soybean sprouts, wax, white)
Lettuce (Boston [Bibb], cos [romaine] iceberg, loose-leaf)
Lotus root
Mushrooms
Mustard greens
Okra
Onions
Parsley
Parsnips
Peas (see also *legumes*)

Peppers (green, hot chili—green
    and red, red)
Pimientos
Potatoes
Pumpkins
Radishes
Rutabaga
Shallots
Spinach

Squash (summer, winter)
Sweet potatoes
Turnips
Water chestnuts
Watercress
Yams
Torula
Zucchini

BREADS

Corn tortillas
Crackers (whole-grain)

Whole-grain bread and rolls
Whole-wheat matzo

CEREALS

Dry flakes (whole grain)
Farina
Granola (unsugared)

Hot cereal (whole-grain)
Millet
Shredded wheat

GRAINS

Barley
Buckwheat (whole-grain)
Corn
Corn field (whole-grain)
Corn grits

Oats, oatmeal
Popcorn (popped)
Rye (whole-grain)
Wheat (whole-grain)

PASTA

Any whole-grain

RICE

Brown
Long-grain

Wild

FRUITS

Acerola (Barbados cherries)
Apples
Apricots
Bananas
Blackberries
Blueberries
Boysenberries
Cantaloupe
Casaba melons

Cherries
Crab apples
Cranberries
Currants
Dates
Elderberries
Figs
Gooseberries
Granadilla (passion fruit)

Grapefruits
Grapes (American, European,
    Thompson seedless)
Guava
Honeydew melons
Kumquats
Lemons
Limes
Litchis
Loganberries
Loquats
Mangos
Nectarines
Oranges
Papayas
Peaches
Pears
Persimmons
Pineapples
Plums
Pomegranates
Prickly pears
Quinces
Raspberries
Rhubarb
Strawberries
Tangelos
Tangerines
Watermelons

Lean-Source Protein: The Stuff Dreams and Bodies Are Made Of

Americans eat the wrong proteins and far too much of them. In the past eighty years we've gone from a country that consumed most of its protein in the form of nutrient-rich and low-fat grains, cereals and legumes to one that relies on calorie-rich and high-fat meat and dairy products.

To make matters worse, inaccurate common wisdom fools us into consuming about twice as much protein as we require. "If protein is that important," the reasoning goes, "what could be wrong with more?" Plenty, as it happens.

Let's begin at our favorite place; the beginning. Just what is protein? What roles does it play in nourishing the body?

Carbohydrates and fats are composed of three simple elements: carbon, hydrogen and oxygen. Add nitrogen to the mix and you can create tiny molecules called amino acids, twenty-two varieties of which may be found in living cells. These building blocks can be strung together in an almost infinite number of ways to create an almost infinite types of protein. The uses of protein in your body are as numerous as the types of proteins that exist. A few of the more important functions proteins perform are:

71

- the structure of muscle, bone, cartilage, hair, skin, nails, blood, lymph and blood vessels
- the formation of antibodies to resist disease
- the delivery of oxygen and nutrients to your cells through the bloodstream.

Of the twenty-two amino acids we require, all but nine can be produced by the body itself. The others, which must be obtained through dietary intake, are called the essential amino acids.

Most animal proteins—that is, the ones that are found in meats, fish, poultry, dairy products and eggs—contain all nine essential amino acids and varying amounts of the nonessential ones. They are thus known as complete proteins. Proteins found in vegetable and legume sources are called incomplete, for they lack sufficient amounts of one or more of the essential amino acids. With the proper guidance, however, plant protein sources combined *within a single meal* can complement each other, and all twenty-two amino acids may be supplied. For obvious reasons, this combination of sources is called complementary protein.

If you choose to forego animal sources of protein entirely, you can still obtain *all* of the necessary amino acids by combining the right incomplete proteins from vegetable sources within one meal. Follow these guidelines:

- Combine legumes (see the list of vegetable sources of fiber, pages 69–70) with corn, rice, wheat, sesame seeds, barley or oats.
- Combine rice with wheat, legumes or sesame seeds.
- Combine wheat with either legumes or soybean/legume mixes (e.g., soybeans and peanuts).

Many societies around the world complement incomplete plant proteins with small amounts of complete animal proteins. Pastas with meat or meat sauce and stir-fried rice with meat or seafood are fine examples of this strategy.

As important as how you choose your protein is when and how much you consume. Protein cannot be stored by the body; it must be consumed, in small quantities, at every meal. And, perhaps not coincidentally, the stress on your digestive and endocrine organs is significantly lessened by taking your protein in five or six small meals—just the advice we gave you to stabilize hunger and minimize calorie overflow and fat storage. (Everything is starting to fall into place now, isn't it? We told you we'd order your universe!) Eat too much protein and the excess nitrogen that must be eliminated in the urine can potentially stress the kidneys. Excess protein consumption can also reduce body levels of calcium. And of course any excess calories you consume will eventually find their metabolic way into storage as body fat, an effect far from the one you expect or want protein to achieve.

Complete or complementary proteins must be consumed at *each* meal, but the required amounts will surely surprise you. Human protein needs are at their absolute highest in infants—a less-than-awesome one gram of protein per pound of body weight. Your requirements decline rather steadily as you age, and although they are higher than normal for pregnant and nursing women and athletes, they never exceed one gram per pound of ideal body weight. The amount of protein you require is determined by your lean body mass—your total body weight minus stored fat; a 170-pound man can fulfill his entire daily protein requirement with the following meager portions: one three-ounce pork chop, a quarter of a cup of cottage cheese and three ounces of tuna.

The Tale of Dietary Fat

But we still haven't told you the *whole* story: why we've coded your protein as lean-source.

Despite a multitude of uses within the body, fat has been identified as the number-one dietary villain. Fat has been linked with varying degrees of scientific certainty to coronary artery disease and cancers of the colon, breast and uterus. The general overconsumption of fat, and its link to obesity, is similarly felt to cause disorders of the liver and kidneys and play a role in the development of arthritis, back pain, diabetes, gout and sexual dysfunction. So why eat fat at all?

The primary reason is the "essential fatty acid" linolenic acid. It is found mostly in polyunsaturated fats, which the body requires for synthesis of other important fats. An adult's linolenic acid requirement is met by about one to two percent of their daily calories, or 30 to 60 calories' worth of vegetable oil for an active male. It's the other functions of fat, however, that raise an acceptable daily intake to about 20 to 25 percent of your caloric total only about *half* of what most Americans now consume in their daily diets.

Fats serve to make foods taste better, satisfy your appetite and, as the most slowly digested nutrient, delay the onset of hunger. They also transport the four vitamins that are soluble *only* in fat—A, D, E and K.

It's not fat in general that has been linked to disease, but a particular type, for which humans have no specific requirement. We're speaking, of course, about saturated fat.

The 1,000 or so milligrams of cholesterol produced by the liver each day are absolutely essential to normal physiological function. Cell membranes, nerve fiber myelin sheaths, vitamin D and sex hormone production all depend upon cholesterol. It is the 600 or more milligrams that you add each day through dietary intake, the type of fat you consume, and your individual response to stress that are the straws that break the camel's back (and give the camel heart disease or cancer, as well). And take note: cholesterol is found *only* in animal protein tissues, such as muscle, fat and organs, and in some dairy products, such as whole milk and eggs.

As we have mentioned, it may be the *kind* of fat, rather than the amount of exogenous, or dietary, cholesterol you consume, that affects your health. Levels of blood cholesterol, which correlate well with heart disease, tend to be elevated by high dietary levels of saturated fat consumption and lowered by substitution of polyunsaturated fat for some saturated fat. Such a strategy of change in fat consumption is now supported by hard medical research. A ten-year, $150 million study of 3,806 men by the National Heart, Lung, and Blood Institute, released in early 1984, tightened what is thought to be the last screw in the cholesterol–heart disease link.

Researchers showed conclusively that the use of the cholesterol-lowering prescription drug cholestyramine was able to decrease the rate of coronary deaths by 24 percent, and the rate of nonfatal heart attacks by 19 percent. Since drug therapy is recommended only for those in the highest blood-cholesterol category, dietary modifications such as the cholesterol-lowering switch from saturated to polyunsaturated fats are the strategy of choice.

The chemical difference between saturates and polyunsaturates* has a visible effect: As the fat molecules fill up with hydrogen atoms, they begin to harden at room temperature. Keep these visual clues in mind when you're making food choices. Animal fats, like butter or lard, which have a high percentage of saturated fats, are solid at room temperature, while vegetable fats, which are predominantly *un*saturated (with the exception of palm and coconut oils, which are highly saturated), are almost always liquid at room temperature. As a matter of fact, you'll rarely hear anyone refer to vegetable "fats"; they commonly speak of vegetable oils.

So far so good. Diets high in saturated fats tend to raise blood cholesterol; diets high in polyunsaturated fats tend to lower it. There is even a simple ratio you can use to judge the acceptability of a product: If the manufacturer's label tells you the amounts of polyunsaturated (P) and saturated (S) fats present, the P to S ratio should be at least 2:1. A 100-percent pure vegetable oil (safflower,

---

* There is room for at least four additional hydrogen atoms per molecule in polyunsaturated fats, and no room, or saturation, in saturated fats. Some fats, such as peanut and olive oils and margarine are monosaturated, with room for two additional hydrogen. These fats are considered to be unsaturated.

sunflower seed and corn oils are good examples) may contain 9 grams of polyunsaturates and 2 grams of saturates per tablespoon, a highly favorable ratio of 9:2, or 4.5:1. And it contains no cholesterol.

Cholesterol is carried in the blood by three major compounds, called lipoproteins. These fat-protein substances are believed to have very different effects on coronary heart-disease risk, and are themselves affected by dietary cholesterol intake.

The apparently "good" form, called HDL for high-density lipoprotein, seems to reduce the risk of heart disease by removing cholesterol deposits from artery walls (arterio- or atherosclerosis) and transporting them to the liver for eventual safe disposal. It also appears that polyunsaturated fats, such as the vegetable oils described above, favor the effects of HDLs and decrease the effects of the other two lipoproteins, LDL (low-density) and VLDL (very low-density lipoprotein). Production of these latter two cholesterol carriers, which make up about 70 percent of total cholesterol, is stimulated by the consumption of saturated animal fats.

Strenuous aerobic exercise (of which running is the most effective form) also seems to raise HDL levels. Caution is advised here, however, since the mileage levels required to raise HDLs may be far in excess of what is needed for optimal fitness and what is safe for your musculoskeletal system. This very hot topic of overload will get major attention in the Quantum Exercise chapter, but actually holds a lesson or two for us here.

Just as an overload of protein, vitamins or saturated fats may be hazardous, recent research suggests that *unusually* high intakes of polyunsaturated fats may be physiologically dangerous. However, *judicious* replacement of saturated fats with polyunsaturated fats offers little or no risk.

The following table offers some sensible and easy-to-follow guidelines for decreasing your consumption of saturated fats. The list that follows it offers you a wide choice of lean-source proteins.

Quantum Guidelines to Dietary Fat Moderation

Substitute these items:
- Highly polyunsaturated vegetable oil (such as Puritan® oil) and margarine
- Fish, poultry and veal
- Skim milk
- Skim milk cheeses, uncreamed or low-fat cottage cheese
- ice milk and sherbet

For these items:
- Lard, meat fat, shortening and butter
- Beef, lamb and pork
- Whole milk and cream
- Whole milk cheeses and creamed cottage cheese
- ice cream.

Do:
- Select lean meat and lean cuts of meat
- Trim away excess fat from meat before cooking
- Buy only ground beef that is prepared from lean meat.

Limit your intake of:
- Egg yolks
- Shellfish
- Bacon, sausage, cold cuts and organ meats (like liver)
- Chocolate and "rich" desserts.

Table courtesy of Procter & Gamble Co., Cincinnati, Ohio

LEANSOURCE PROTEINS

Poultry (with skin and excess fat removed)
Chicken
Cornish hen
Dove
Duck
Goose
Grouse
Guinea fowl
Hazel hen
Partridge
Pheasant
Pigeon
Prairie chicken
Quail
Snipe
Squab
Turkey
Woodcock

Meat:
Veal
Dairy:
Buttermilk (from skim milk)
Low-fat cottage cheese
Low-fat milk (1% milk fat)
Low-fat yogurt
Nonfat dry milk
Skim-milk cheeses
Skim milk
Skim-milk-and-banana shake
Fish and Shellfish:
Abalone
Alewife
Anchovies
Barracuda
Bass (black sea, largemouth, smallmouth, striped, white)
Bluefish

Buffalo fish
Bullhead, black
Butterfish (northern, Gulf)
Carp
Catfish
Chub
Clams
Cod
Crab
Crappie (white)
Crayfish
Croaker (Atlantic, white, yellowfin)
Cusk
Drum (red [redfish])
Flounder
Fluke
Frog legs
Grouper
Haddock
Hake (including whiting)
Halibut (Atlantic, California,
    Greenland, Pacific)
Kingfish
Lake herring
Lingcod
Lobster (northern, spiny)
Muskellunge
Mussels (Atlantic, Pacific)

Ocean perch (Pacific)
Octopus
Oysters (eastern)
Perch (ocean [redfish, rosefish],
    yellow)
Pickerel
Pike (blue, northern, walleye)
Plaice
Pollack
Porgy (scup)
Redhorse
Rockfish
Rosefish (ocean perch)
Sablefish
Salmon (chum, silver [coho],
    sockeye)
Skate
Snails
Snapper (red, gray)
Sole
Swordfish
Tautog (blackfish)
Tilefish
Tomcod (Atlantic)
Tuna (albacore, bluefin, yellowfin)
Turbot
Turtle (green)
Whitebait

Clear Water: Life's Most Precious Fluid

No substance is more abundant on planet Earth or in our bodies than water. Composing 70 percent of our bodily substance, water is involved in all functions of our cells, organs and systems. From its more obvious roles in forming the bases of blood, lymph, saliva, mucus and digestive juices, to its unsuspected but essential role in allowing carbon dioxide and oxygen to dissolve and diffuse across the microscopic membranes deep within our lungs, water must be ranked as our most critical nutrient. Humans have been known to live without carbohydrates, fats and proteins for a month or more, but we will die in a matter of days if deprived of water.

Water is important enough to have an access code all to itself; but for all its importance, we take water for granted. We are told time and time again about the value, the *need*, for at least eight eight-ounce glasses of clear water each day, but our sixty-four-ounce liquid fix has come by way of coffee, tea, milk, soft drinks and juices. (There is nothing wrong with the occasional soft drink, cup of coffee or tea, provided you fulfill your body's need for clear water.) But your involvement in *Quantum Fitness* suggests a willingness to change, a mental readiness to work on the Quantum goals of health, performance and longevity.

Where is this precious fluid best obtained? Your local health department or water-supply office periodically tests drinking water and is your first information stop. Many areas still benefit from clean, clear, tasty water. Your alternatives, should local water supplies be in any way tainted or too "soft" (a condition that is now being linked to heart disease), are filtration or bottled water. Although neither option is without problems, both can provide you with relief from the shortcomings of your local water-supply.*

Your best bet in bottled waters are unprocessed spring waters from areas that are far removed from industrial pollutants. Mineral contents vary, depending on the geographic locations of the water sources, and should be researched if you are on a sodium-restricted diet.

YOUR QUANTUM NUTRITION PROGRAM

The Quantum Nutrition codes establish the boundaries for your individual dietary strategy. By using the three Quantum access codes—fiber-based carbohydrates, lean-source proteins and clear water—we've spared you the food exchanges, portion-measuring

---

* The well-respected publication *Consumer Reports* has devoted much attention recently to the effectiveness of home filtration systems. Comments and ratings appeared in the February, June and July 1983 issues.

and calorie-counting of other regimens. Ideally you will include lean-source protein and fiber-based carbohydrates at every meal, and drink sixty-four ounces (again, eight eight-ounce glasses) of clear water every day. The program may not differ greatly from your current eating habits, but will put new emphasis on variety. Your schedule allowing, you will consume smaller and more frequent meals. Your snacks will include fruits and vegetables, although variety and rotational selection of foods will allow the occasional ice-cream treat.

But what of the executive or the professional woman/housewife with a career *and* two kids *and* a husband? They can work the same access codes and Quantum principles into their special lifestyles. Mornings are too busy to plan your breakfasts? Why not whip up a tasty and nutritious shake the night before with skim milk, an egg and some fruit? Add a slice of whole-wheat toast and a light swipe of polyunsaturated margarine and you're out of the house in minutes. Big business lunch ahead? You'll be surprised at how accommodating restaurateurs can be if you ask for your fish broiled, not fried, or your salad dressing on the side, or only a small amount of hollandaise sauce. Get some new cookbooks; there's a great trend afoot to cook "quick and healthy." Are you too tired to spend hours preparing dinner? Investigate steaming, a simple way to prepare a broad variety of foods, including fish, lean meats, vegetables and carbohydrate sources. You might try preparing and cooking larger quantities of your favorite dishes on the weekends so that your weeknights will be less hectic.

By applying the following three steps, you will find ways to bring the access codes and Quantum principles to your dining table and integrate them into your daily life.

Step I

Review the lists of foods under the Quantum Nutrition access codes. Select foods from these and other comparable sources for your breakfast, lunch and dinner menus. Base your choices on your own tastes and needs. Do not be bound by habit or tradition: Try broiled fish and rice for breakfast, like the Japanese, or a simple supper of vegetable soup with white beans, whole-wheat bread and fresh fruit, like the French.

Step II

By applying the Quantum principles of variety and rhythmic rotation, you will assure optimum nutrient availability of vitamins, minerals and fiber in addition to your protein, carbohydrate and basic fat needs.

Try not to eat the same foods every day. If chicken is your favorite lean-source protein, try to eat it no more than every third day.

Step III

Quantum Nutrition simulation cycles are the final step to assuring an ongoing state of positive adaptation. You will read, control and direct the signals that your body and mind are continually sending through the power of your simulation cycles. You now have the means to construct your individualized plan no matter who you are or what your specific goals may be. Abiding by the codes, remaining flexible and timely in your choices of foods and applying the appropriate simulations will make the Quantum nutritional plan a part of your life.

FOOD FOR THOUGHT: QUANTUM NUTRITION SIMULATIONS

The best way to ensure success in your nutrition and weight-control program is to combine Quantum mental- and Nutrition access codes. This means using adaptive relaxation and simulation, self-talk cycles to reinforce your use of fiber-based carbohydrates, lean-source protein and clear water on a daily basis.

The first step is to use the autogenic training exercises you learned in Chaper Two to induce passive relaxation. You should practice warming your arms, legs and stomach; cooling your forehead; relaxing your breathing; and slowing down your heartbeat at least once every day for about fifteen minutes. Continue this daily practice until you can bring about the desired passive relaxation state in a matter of minutes.

Entering this passive or adaptive relaxation state will help your management of stress by reducing the effects of internal and environmental factors that result in chronic overeating. The adaptive relaxation state is the ideal time for you to verbalize, visualize and emotionalize the positive self-talk simulations for your unique, specific nutritional enhancement.

Here are some general suggested self-talk statements to help set up your Quantum leap in nutrition. Construct your own specific statements and use them every day.

> "I am in control of my eating habits."
> "I eat a nutritious breakfast every day."
> "I eat small portions of nutritious food when I'm hungry."
> "I eat fresh vegetables, whole grain and fresh fruit every day."
> "I enjoy small portions of skinless chicken, turkey or fish as my protein."
> "My Quantum nutrition codes are fiber-based carbohydrates, lean-source proteins and clear water."
>
> "When I'm thirsty, I usually drink clear water."
> "I drink at least one glass of clear water with every meal."
> "I enjoy sparkling water as a social drink."
> "Water is my favorite fitness drink."
>
> "My food is naturally salty."
> "I seldom eat dessert, but when I do, usually it is fresh fruit."
> "I eat slowly and chew each bite thoroughly."
> "I take small bites of food and place my fork or spoon on my plate between bites."
> "I eat only when I'm hungry and only for my good health."
> "I like and respect myself and I eat what's best for me."

"I look slim and attractive in by bathing suit."
"When I am window-shopping I like the reflection of me I
 see."
"I weigh [your desired weight] pounds and feel great."
"I am a strong person."
"I'm happy being me right now."

Since you are human, there will be moments when you will stray off the Quantum Nutrition path. It may be over the holidays. It could be on a vacation. It may be on any Saturday. Those are the times when a Quantum individual utilizes positive-feedback self-talk. Also, as you are progressing on this lifetime-fitness journey there will be those who will compliment you and a few who may try to rain on your nutrition parade.

Your feedback self-talk is just as important as your feedforward or affirmation self-talk. In response to any criticism about your progress, your mental and verbal response should be: "Slowly but surely it's working for me. I can feel the benefits."

When you have given in to the temptations of the menu, the wine list and the French-pastry cart, your feedback should be: "Because of my daily nutrition habits I can enjoy this rare occasion."

When you are sitting with the remnants of a fast-food splurge, rather than berate yourself and feel guilty, your self-talk might be: "Come on, I deserve better fuel than this. This is not like me. Next time I'll say no!"

And when anyone tells you how good you look or pays you any compliment at any time, for any reason, your unhesitating reply should be: "Thank you. I really appreciate that, coming from you."

This is the self-talk of a winner. This is the vocabulary of the Quantum You. Now you're ready for action!

QUANTUM EXERCISE

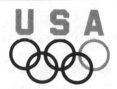

IN THE Olympian quest for health, peak performance and longevity, it is Quantum Nutrition that fuels your hidden potential and Quantum Exercise that unlocks it.

The same Quantum principles that direct your mental and nutritional action plans very much explain and enable the strategies that are Quantum Exercise. Through variety you will satisfy the diverse needs of your body, avoid the overtraining syndrome and maintain a healthy and vibrant interest in exercise. Through adaptation you will understand that rest and recovery are as important to fitness as exercise itself. Through rhythm you will learn to tune in to your body's internal language and to create a dynamically balanced approach to fitness that is yours alone.

Utilizing the access codes of core balance, rhythmic endurance and multijoint patterning exercise, your fitness program will be far more than an exercise prescription written by some outsider. You will learn to understand your body's rhythms and become an integral part of your own fitness program.

MIND OVER MUSCLES

We have some good news and some bad news. During this century, technology has advanced at an astounding rate. Those of us in industrialized countries have radically reshaped the environment in which we live. We have changed from a fundamentally physically oriented, rural-based society into a population of harried city and suburb dwellers who pay more attention to maintaining the condition of our cars and our pets than we devote to our own health. As brain power is taking over from brawn, so have technical devices and gadgets assumed an increasing amount of work formerly performed by muscle power.

Elevators and escalators have replaced stairways, automation has outmoded perspiration and the hand-pushed lawn mower is as obsolete as the horse-drawn carriage. In our quest to make our existence more bearable, we have been successful in reducing the amount of human effort and human energy expended. We have conserved our energy and saved our physical effort for our leisure-time activities. In the process, we have become fat and sedentary, occupying most of our free hours watching our favorite heroes and heroines being active on the television screen. We have become a nation of spectators instead of participants.

But you are different. You have decided to break away from the pack. While you don't take yourself so seriously that you have become preoccupied only with muscle tone, you are involved in a continuing self-management program to achieve physical and emotional excellence. For you, fitness is your way of life and it is in your life to stay.

As you read this chapter on Quantum Exercise, remember the Quantum Force: When your mind talks, your body listens. Getting in shape and staying in shape is a matter of mind over muscles. World-class athletes generally concur that once they are in physical condition and have mastered the basic skills, 70 to 90 percent of the outcome is determined by mental factors.

To enjoy the maximum performance from your body in today's fast-lane environment, devote at least as much effort to your autogenic adaptive relaxation, visualization and self-talk simulation training as you do to your physical exercise routines. The difference between the average individual and the Quantum You is the mental edge. Thousands of athletes function well in many day-to-day situations and occasionally during high-level competition. At a critical point in their competitive careers, however, they are unable to perform, because the psychological skills needed to complement their physical expertise have not been developed to the same degree. Among athletes this is referred to as "choking."

Those elite athletes who have developed advanced psychological skills usually have done so through years of sports competition. Veteran athletes often recognize that experience has taught them valuable lessons in strategy and psychology. Their physical tools had been sharpened early in their athletic careers, but only as they developed adaptive relaxation, visualization and self-talk simulation skills did they become members of the elite. Ironically, by the time some athletes have developed these mental skills through trial and error their physical abilities have begun to decline. As one former world-class track star said, "By the time I finally learned that it was mind over muscles, my muscles didn't care anymore."

USING THE QUANTUM FORCE IN EXERCISE

Assessment

The first step in entering an exercise program is a comprehensive analysis of your current fitness level. This profile should include:

- a complete physical examination by your physician
- a fitness evaluation at a professional clinic or fitness center (which may include a stress test if you are over thirty-five years of age and have one or more risk factors, such as obesity or smoking)
- a personal inventory of your exercise likes and dislikes and the things that have or haven't worked for you in the past (for example, you may not be a swimmer, but you enjoy bicycling every chance you get)
- an honest, personal evaluation of your mental, emotional, nutritional and physical well-being.

Goals

Goals are the engines that power our lives, and written goals are the tools that make fitness possible. Successful individuals have game plans and programs that are clearly defined and to which they constantly refer. The reason that most people never reach their fitness goals is that they never really took the time to set them in the first place.

First, set long-range goals that have some exciting pull for you, then set short-term goals that are just beyond your current levels of strength and endurance. If your pulse rate hovers in the eighties when you are resting, set your immediate sights on bringing it down to seventy-nine. Yes, we know that Frank Shorter's resting pulse is normally in the thirties; you can make that a long-term goal if you like. But be realistic: If you want to lose twenty-five pounds by the end of the year, fine. Your short-term goal can be a weight loss of two to five pounds per month.

We have found that it is critically important to use an incremental approach to fitness. Many individuals drop out of exercise programs and diet regimens because they expect immediate results. They try their hardest but feel that they can't measure up to the standards their role models achieve. They want positive feedback, but all they feel are aches and pains.

By setting goals that are relatively easy to achieve, it is easier to keep on track and get back on track if necessary. The achievement of incremental goals gives you confidence and is reinforcement toward staying with the program until you've reached your long-range goals. Every Olympic decathlon winner in the last twenty years has said that stair-stepping their goals over a period of time was one of the keys to their success. What works for them can work for you!

Data Acquisition

The concepts and information you will find in this book are just the beginning of your reeducation. There are hundreds of worthwhile books and articles published on mental and physical fitness; you can start with the ones on our reading list. Attend lectures, seminars or workshops, and take advantage of the wealth of knowledge now available on cassettes. Make your car into a mobile university!

If you're striving to improve your performance in a particular sport, consider taking instruction, either group or private, from the best sources you can find.

Adaptive Relaxation

Prior to your regular exercise routine, get into the habit of using your autogenic training to warm your arms, legs and stomach. Using verbal self-talk and visualization; check to make sure that your breathing is relaxed and effortless and that your heartbeat is slow and regular. As you exercise, learn to listen to your pulse rate with your inner ear. As you rest and recover after your exercise program, use autogenic mental exercise to relax and bring your heartbeat back to its normal resting rate. The ability of the mind to learn to listen to the body talk is remarkable; it is being used effectively by our Olympic pistol and rifle competitors to squeeze the trigger between heartbeats for the highest number of bull's-eyes!

Simulation

Valeri Borzov, the great Russian sprinter, is remembered by fans throughout the world as winner of the one-hundred- and two-hundred-meter track events at the 1972 Munich Olympic Games. In an interview after the Munich Games, Borzov described his mental state during his winning one-hundred-meter performance:

> As I placed my feet against the starting blocks I began to run the race in my mind. The spectators, naturally, could not know this. They only saw Borzov walk up slowly to the starting line, carefully place his feet against the starting blocks and freeze in that pose until the command "Ready!" Mentally, though, I was somewhat ahead of that. I was already running. By learning to draw a mental picture of the race while I was still at the starting line, I was able to react to the starting shot with split-second speed. And when the shot was fired, my inner robot—programmed to get me out of the motionless state—switched on and took over.

By using the Quantum access codes of adaptive relaxation and simulation, you, too, can run ahead of the pack. When you wake up in the morning, use general and specific self-talk, feedforward simulation: "I am strong and full of energy. . . . Today is my best day ever. . . . I can feel my body is more healthy now. . . . I enjoy exercise and physical activity. . . . I'm a winner. . . . I like who I see in the mirror. . . ."

As you warm up prior to your regular exercise routine, visualize yourself measuring your pulse at a certain rate during aerobic exercise and then noticing it recover to your normal rate within a specified period of time. After your exercise routine or after high-level performance, use self-talk feedback simulation to reinforce a positive self-image about your fitness progress: "That was a good workout. . . . I can feel the progress and the benefits. . . . My recovery rate is faster now. . . . I can improve that performance. . . . That's not like me. I will do better next time. . . . I can see the vitality and positive change when I look in the mirror. . . .

While you are walking, jogging or engaged in any form of physical exercise, visualize yourself as that person you would most like to become. See your trim and muscled body. Feel your vitality and energy. Experience the joy and exhilaration of your higher performance levels.

You *can* take charge. Your mind can make the impossible possible—then actual.

QUANTUM PRINCIPLES AND EXERCISE

Variety: Avoiding Too Much of a Good Thing

We cannot stress too strongly that lack of variety is one of the major stumbling blocks along the bumpy road to fitness. Somewhere along the way you lost *mental* flexibility and got locked into jogging or weight-lifting or some other less-than-complete form of exercise. You lost sight of the fact that our wonderfully complex bodies can move in wonderfully complex ways; that fitness means coordinating muscles and limbs, which are capable of an infinite variety of effective movements; that the body must be continually challenged with a wide variety of physical tasks or it will cease to grow. Just as variety in food choices can ensure satisfaction of the body's nutrient needs, variety in exercise can satisfy the body's requirements for movement.

We have identified two other areas in which attention to variety will nourish the Quantum Fitness approach. The exercise dropout, an all-too-common sight in front of the television screens of America these days, most likely got bored with his focused attack on fitness. No one told him that, properly orchestrated, running, swimming, cycling, skating and jumping rope can all work harmoniously and effectively together. He just doesn't know that, way down deep in the cells of his body, where the biofires of fitness burn, the *type* of activity doesn't really matter. Variety may very well have kept him interested and active.

Finally, there's the nemesis of overuse, the repetitive and relentless beating the body takes from a single-minded approach to exercise. Running has a place in fitness. Too much running doesn't. It can manifest itself in any number of ways: fatigue, injury and even certain diseases. Overuse can be entirely avoided if you are willing and able to listen to your body's warnings and allow positive adaptation to take place.

Adaptation: Working with, Not Against, the Body

The Quantum You will listen to the feedback signals of adaptation and will feedforward the structure of your fitness program so that challenges to the body are followed by periods of sufficient rest. Given the nourishment of varied movements and sufficient rest intervals, the body will grow toward heightened efficiency. Abused with overloads of any type—exercise, food or stress—the body will maladapt. Only your own body can tell you when you reach the point of adaptation. Only you can determine when your body has sufficiently renewed itself from the stress of exercise to begin again.

Feedback on the adaptation process is surprisingly plentiful. It's up to *you* to take the time to look for it, understand it and use it. We'd like you to start by using the signals below to monitor your current exercise program. Once you develop a feel for "body talk," you'll be ready to start customizing your own exercise routine.

Given the opportunity to meet the demands you place on it, the body will be glad to respond with these adaptations and more:

- increased aerobic capacity—the ability to work at less than maximal output for long periods of time
- increased anaerobic power—the ability to produce a great amount of work in a short period of time
- increased muscular strength
- improved flexibility

- lowered risk of cardiovascular disease
- improved tolerance of psychological stress
- improved control of body weight through increased metabolic rate as well as increased caloric expenditure
- improved posture and prevention of back pain through balanced strength and mobility of key muscles and joints.

These are the signs that you'll need to determine readiness for another stress/adaptation cycle:

- **Pulse rate.** The morning pulse rate, taken upon awakening, is an excellent indicator of overtraining and physical distress. Our Olympic coaches and athletes keep close watch on the morning pulse rate and ease up on training when it is significantly higher than normal. Your pulse rate during exercise will be your tool for applying the access code of rhythmic endurance; you'll learn more about that shortly.
- **Sleep.** One's nightly sleep is considered a critically important adaptation period. Any changes in the duration or quality of the night's sleep, or the ease of falling asleep, may indicate overtraining and insufficient rest.
- **Unusual weight loss.** The stress of overtraining is often reflected in unusual or unexpected drops in body weight.
- **Excessive or unusual thirst.**
- **General fatigue.** Insufficient rest may manifest itself by general feelings of lethargy and malaise.
- **Loss of rhythm during exercise.** When movement elegance or form is faltering, the body is asking for a chance to rest, recover and recharge. Along with exercise pulse rate, this is one of the best signs that the body is ready for a short rest.
- **Excessive pain.** If you have pain, you should have stopped already.

Rhythm: Marching to the Biological Beat

Rhythm is the governing principle of Quantum *balance* in your exercise strategy. Listening to the biological language of adaptation—pulse rate, sleep, hunger, thirst—will encourage you to cre-

93

ate your own unique exercise rhythm. Your Quantum Exercise program depends wholly upon the body's acceptance of physical stress. When you read readiness, you exercise. When you read fatigue, overwork or distress, you rest.

The Quantum You will go beyond day-to-day rhythms of rest and exercise. You will learn to read the moment-to-moment rhythms *within* exercise as reflected by your heart rate response; and bring the concept of stress and adaptation to each exercise in your program.

We also recommend that you time your exercise sessions to coincide with your daily highs in body temperature. Our Olympic Chronobiology Project at Harvard University is relating the daily flows of several physiological rhythms to muscular strength. You can tap into one of these rhythms at home with a thermometer. Plot your body temperature at two-to-four-hour intervals for several days. You may be surprised to find that your personal daily highs and lows match the temperature swings quite closely. Train at peak times for peak training gains.

Armed with this new knowledge of variety, adaptation and rhythm in exercise, you are ready to learn the access codes.

THE QUANTUM EXERCISE ACCESS CODES

Fitness Synergies: A Quantum Approach

No one would argue that the individual atoms that combine to form your body possess any life force. They are simply structures of electrons, protons and neutrons. Yet, somehow, in their combination to form your bodily substance, they produce life. This synergism—the whole being greater than the sum of the parts—is no less true of the combination of access codes in each of our middle three Olympic rings. The three Quantum access codes for exercise—pelvic balance, rhythmic endurance and multijoint patterning exercise—are the final mini-synergism before your Quantum leap.

A dynamically balanced exercise program will set off a chain of beneficial physiological and metabolic effects. A proper warmup will allow more mobility and flexibility, which will in turn prepare the body for optimum pelvic balance, rhythmic endurance and multijoint movements. Feedback-guided, rhythmic and multijoint exercises will take the body to its safe limits of stress and will cause a chain reaction of positive adaptations in muscle, bone and connective tissue, cardiovascular function, hormone systems and neurological patterning, which in turn will bring you closer to your Quantum goals of health, peak performance and longevity.

Applying the Access Codes

In applying the three Quantum exercise access codes, you'll need to keep the following points in mind:

• **Overuse is abuse.** A crash exercise program is no more effective than a crash diet, and is probably more dangerous. You stand to gain nothing from a headlong rush into exercise, and have everything to lose. The Quantum You is mentally ready for a gradual and intelligent approach to lifetime fitness. Listen to your body and add exercise stress in acceptable amounts.

Use your pulse. Many of the decisions you make about your exercise program will hinge on your heart rate. As the most effective window to your body's metabolism, it will enable you to create, rather than follow, workout strategies. That's why this book does not contain page after page of workouts. Guidelines in the form of the access codes will set the boundaries and specify the conditions of your sessions. *You* will be the architect of your exercise program.

Since the heart rate is an immediate and accurate source of physiological feedback, we advise that it be monitored through all phases of your workouts. The pulse may be simply taken at either the radial artery in the wrist or the carotid artery in the neck. Using the middle three fingers and only light pressure, locate the pulse on the thumb side of the wrist (next to the wiry tendons) or along the windpipe. You can obtain an approximate pulse rate in 10 or 15 seconds by multiplying your resulting count by 6 or 4, respectively.

Recent technological advances have enabled the development of portable pulse-rate monitors. The simplest of these devices reads the heart rate through sensors that sit on the fingertip or earlobe. Though the point of pulse monitors is to measure heart rate during exercise, many of the devices become inaccurate during active movement.

The type of pulse monitor we prefer to use consists of an elastic chest strap that contains two or three flat surfaces, called electrodes, that read heart rate through direct electrical activity. One highly advanced monitor we use with our Olympic athletes incorporates a tiny transmitter on the chest strap to broadcast heart rate to a wrist-worn pulse display/stopwatch unit.* This wrist unit allows the programming of high and low pulse alarms so that a specific target zone can be set. We find it a wonderful extension of our bodies that provides instantaneous, accurate biofeedback without interrupting the exercise in progress.

Just how will heart-rate response help you structure your workouts? Researchers have determined that you will enjoy optimal training benefits (physiological adaptations) when exercise maintains your pulse in an age- and fitness-specific "target zone." This number, falling roughly between 70 and 85 percent of your maximum heart rate, can be estimated simply by subtracting your age from 220, and multiplying the result by 75. A more personalized method of calculating your target heart rate can be achieved through the Karvonen formula:

* The Amerec 150 Sport Tester® is available from the Amerec Corporation, PO Box 3825, Bellevue, WA 98009.

For several consecutive days,

(1) obtain your resting heart rate upon awakening. Use an average in doing the computations to follow.

(2) If you are just beginning an exercise program, you will need to work at no higher than 70 percent of your maximum capacity: Use 0.7 in the equations below. If you are fit and active, increae the intensity to 85 percent or 0.85.

(3) Insert intensity and resting heart rate (RHR) into this equation:

$$[(220 - \text{your age} - \text{RHR}) \times \text{intensity}] + \text{RHR} = \text{Target Heart Rate}$$

$$[(220 - 40 - 75) \times 0.7] + 75 =$$
$$[(105) \times 0.7] + 75 =$$
$$73.5 + 75 = 148.5 \text{ beats per minute}$$

(4) To obtain your target zone, add and subtract five beats in either direction to your target number. In our example, the target zone would be approximately 144 to 154 beats per minute.

(5) As your fitness level improves, you are likely to see a decrease in your resting heart rate. At this point you may want to inch intensity along from the 70-percent level to the 85-percent level. Substituting these new numbers into the Karvonen equation above will assist in keeping your target zone zeroed in on the body's adaptation process.

(6) Finally, as the Quantum You gains the ability to tune in to your own body's rhythms, you will more effectively tune in to your own target heart rate and elminate the need for a general formula.

You need to warm up and cool down. The warm-up and cooldown are important to your core, rhythmic and multijoint exercise sessions. Feedback guides you through your warm-up, which always *precedes* flexibility and mobility work and will be pulse-monitored. Using either your manually taken pulse or an accurate pulse monitor, your rhythmic warm-up in a walk or easy run might proceed in the following fashion:

- Begin light, low-stress exercise. Walking or running easily with a moderate arm swing is the top choice. Let's say you have a starting pulse of 85.
- Walk or run until your pulse reaches 110. Slow the pace, then resume it when your pulse reaches 100.
- Walk or run until your pulse reaches 120. Slow your pace again to allow the pulse to reach 110.
- Repeat as above until your pulse reaches 130. Slow your pace to allow your pulse to drop to 110 and then continue into your rhythmic workout.

This rhythmic approach ensures that exercise stress is applied gradually and at a pace that the body can adapt to. You should aim for a five-to-ten-minute warm-up and, of course, may adjust the target pulses given above according to your own needs.

You should also monitor your post-exercise cool-down through pulse work. The body must readapt to a static state after exercise; its metabolically active systems should be let down slowly. We suggest light exercise, such as walking, until your pulse drops back to the 90-to-110-beat range.

Other warm-up/cool-down choices? Anything that maximizes the involvement of your five-hundred-plus muscles is fair game, which is why walking is a top choice. Easy jumping jacks, with the legs alternating between side-side and front-back kicks, works well. Cycling is a good lower-body and cardiovascular warm-up, but neglects the torso and arms. Performance of your sport activity itself may at times be a good warm-up or cool-down; swimming is a good example. As long as you begin slowly, watch your pulse and do not take cold muscles and connective tissues further than they're ready to go, you'll be fine.

Maintain flexibility and mobility. Following your warm-up, time spent during recovery intervals between periods of rhythmic exercise may be partially devoted to mobility exercises. These are slow, gentle movements that take your limbs through their ranges of motion. Using low-stress movement patterns will increase the efficiency of working limbs without overstretching and damaging muscles and connective tissues. Since these movements all involve multiple joints and muscles, you'll find them discussed in detail under our third access code, multijoint exercise.

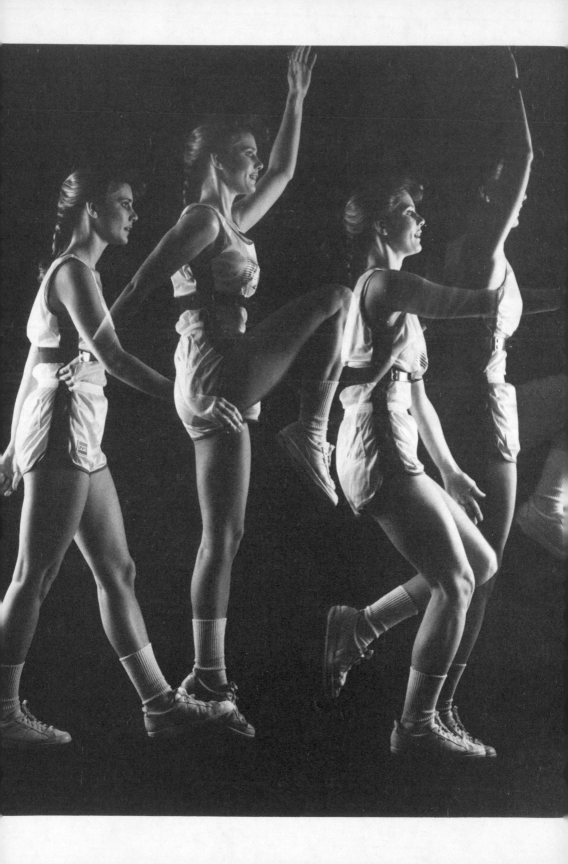

Pelvic Balance: The Foundation for All Movement

Proper balance and posture constitute the foundation from which all effective movements are generated. Balance of the pelvis is the true basis for excellence of movement. Pelvic balance, our first access code, is effective insurance against lower-back disorders, which afflict an estimated eight out of ten American adults.

The pelvis is the supporting platform for the spinal column, anchoring the abdominal and back muscles above, and the thigh muscles (front and back) below and the muscles within the pelvis itself. All of these muscles are crucial to keeping the spinal column in proper alignment as it rests on the pelvis. In order to optimize pelvic balance, the pelvis's flexibility must be maintained. This is largely contingent upon these muscles' being balanced in strength and elasticity. When a group of pelvis-related muscles are weak, shortened or in spasm, the pelvis will lose its stability and flexibility, which can lead to muscular injury or misalignment of the low back, causing back pain.

The purpose of the exercises described in the Pelvic Balance Program below is to restore and/or maintain the functional length and strength of the muscles and balance the pelvis and spinal column. An unbalanced system is the first step to injury.

The Pelvic Balance Program

The following are exercises that will help you to attain dynamic balance.

101

Standing Pelvic Tilt

This exercise works the many internal muscles that control pelvic alignment. It may be performed several times throughout the day.

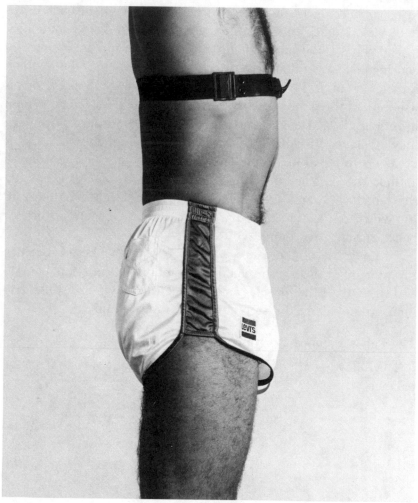

(1) Stand with your feet together, your stomach tucked in, your body straight and your shoulders down.

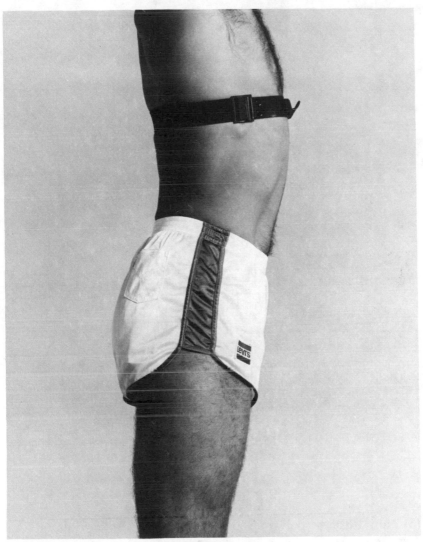

(2) Tilt your pelvis slightly down and backward into a position that adds to the curve of your lower back.

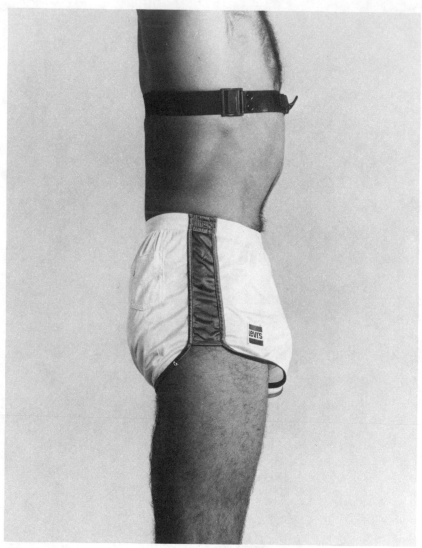

(3) Now tilt your pelvis up and forward. Pull in your abdominal muscles and keep your buttocks tight.

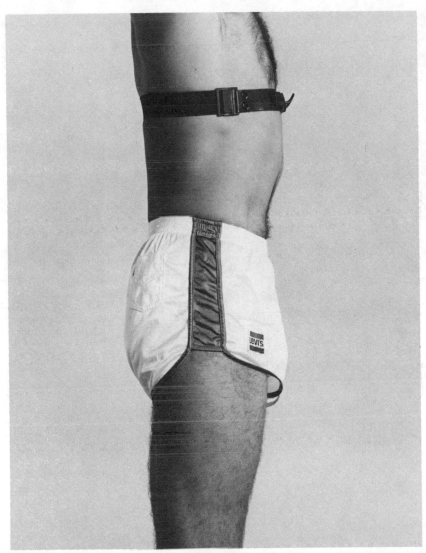

(4) Return to your starting position. This midway position allows optimal alignment of the pelvic girdle, giving the most efficient support to the spinal column and torso.

Pelvic Tilt with Bridge

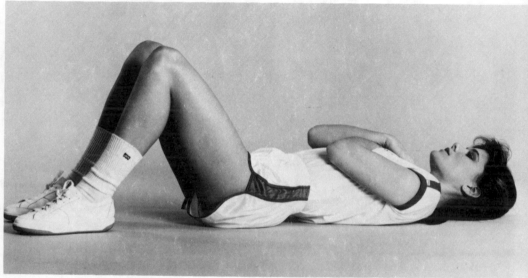

(1) Lie on your back with your arms folded over your chest and your feet placed together a comfortable distance from your buttocks.

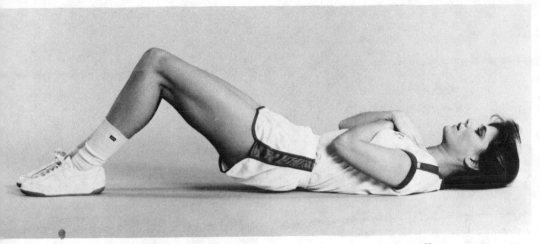

(2) Tilt your pelvis up and forward; your lower back will rise slightly off the floor. This is the same movement you performed in Step 3 of the Standing Pelvic Tilt.

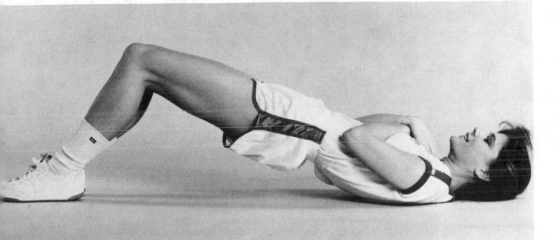

(3) Continue rotating your pelvis forward, using your abdominals and front thigh muscles (quadriceps). Contracting your buttocks will give you an extra boost. Keep your upper back and shoulders on the floor. Hold this position for three seconds and gently lower yourself to the floor.

107

Modified Sit-up with Twist

This is a safe and effective way to strengthen all the abdominal muscles, the *rectus abdominis* and the internal and external obliques. Perform this exercise slowly and rhythmically, pausing between each repetition.

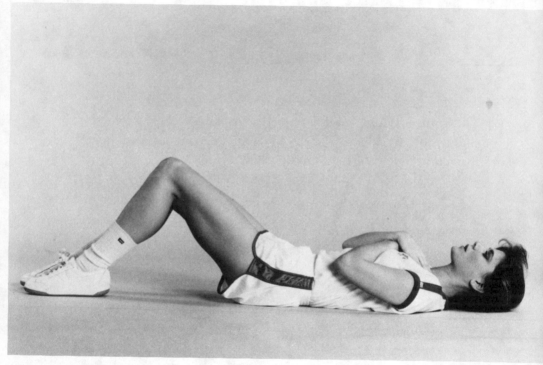

(1) Begin lying on your back with your arms folded over your chest and your feet together a comfortable distance away from your buttocks. The closer your feet are to your buttocks, the more difficult the exercise.

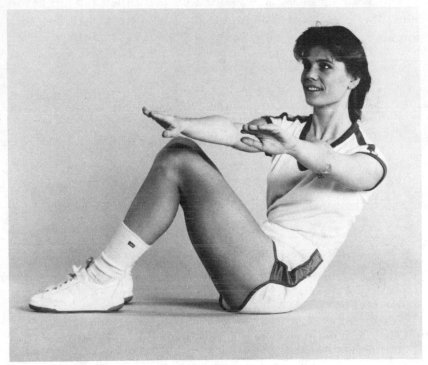

(2) Tuck your chin into your chest and begin to curl up slowly, one vertebrae at a time. Uncross your arms and reach out diagnonally; turn your torso to follow your arms. Curl down, vertebrae by vertebrae, to the floor. Repeat the sit-up, reaching to the opposite side. One sit-up to each side is one repetition of the exercise.

Modified V-up

This is an advanced multijoint sit-up that brings the hip flexors into play. The feet remain on the floor between repetitions; they are *not* held aloft.

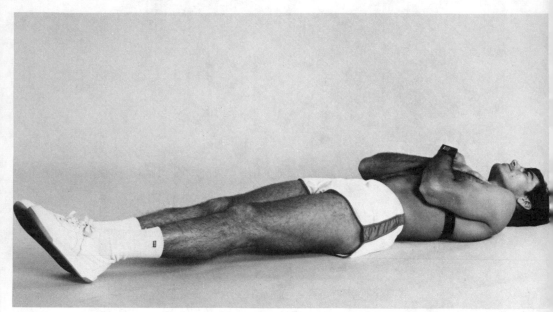

(1) Begin by lying on your back with your legs straight in front of you and your feet together. Cross your arms over your chest.

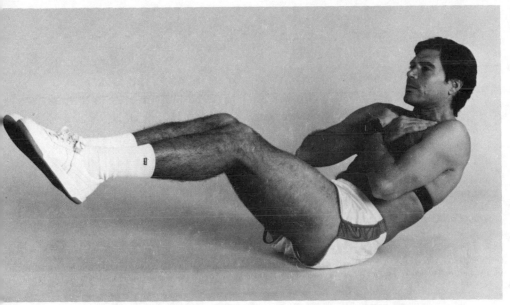

(2) Simultaneously bring your legs to your chest, knees flexed, and curl up your torso, vertebrae by vertebrae.

(3) Continue raising your legs and torso until they meet. Return slowly to your starting position. *Do not hold your feet off the floor in between repetitions.*

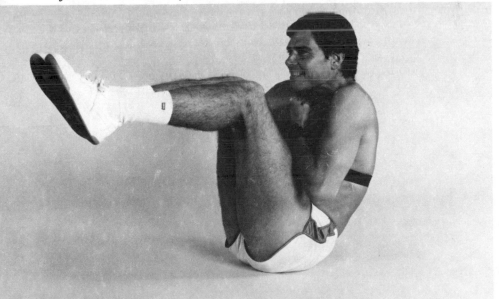

Back Extension—Torso Only

The beginner's version of this exercise involves the torso only. It is an excellent workout for the muscles of the lower back and those along the spinal column. This exercise should be performed slowly and smoothly; the height you attain is not important.

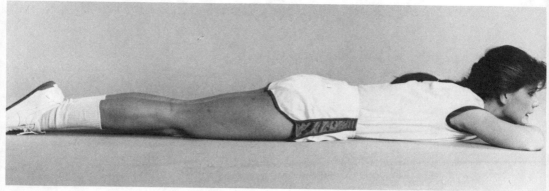

(1) Begin by lying on your stomach with your legs extended. Rest your chin on your folded arms.

(2) Keeping your legs on the floor, begin raising your head from the floor. The neck and torso follow, a vertebrae at a time. *Lift only as high as you can comfortably;* this is not a contest to see who has the highest extension. Hold the extended position for a count of two, then return slowly to your starting position.

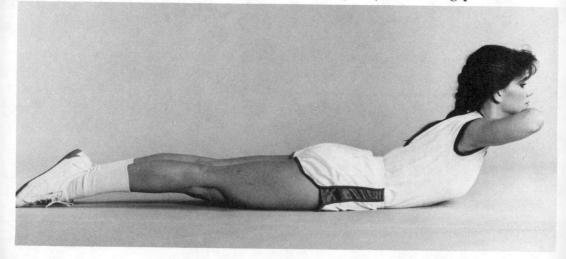

Back Extension with Leg Elevation

The advanced version of the back extension brings the muscles of the buttocks (gluteals) and hamstrings into play. We suggest you master the Back Extension—Torso Only before you move on to this.

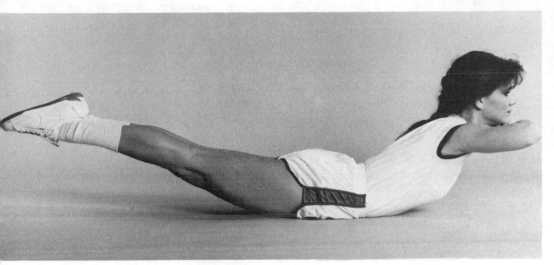

(1) Begin by lying on your stomach with your legs extended. Rest your chin on your folded arms.

(2) Simultaneously raise your torso (as you did in the previous exercise) and your legs. This will require you to contract your buttocks and hamstrings (the muscles in the backs of your thighs). Hold this position for a count of two, release and return your torso and legs slowly to the floor.

113

Squat

This is the most effective exercise we know of to develop pelvic balance, muscular endurance and strength in a large variety of muscles. We will discuss this exercise in greater detail in the section on rhythmic endurance.

Inversion Exercises

We have chosen to include several basic exercises that can be performed on an *oscillating* inversion system using separate ankle holders (gravity boots). Exercising in the inverted position helps you stretch and lengthen key muscles, such as those in the thighs, abdomen, back and pelvis, while simultaneously decompressing the spinal column and joints by using the natural pull of gravity. This exciting concept has unique benefits, and we highly recommend its use. While in an inverted position, remember to keep moving; hanging for extended periods in the stationary position is outside the boundaries of safe use for this device.* The Gravity Guiding System is an important contribution to pelvic balance. These exercises are only a selection from a program that can contribute much to your musculoskeletal integrity and balance.

> **CAUTION:** Patients should seek qualified medical advice before engaging in any exercise program, inversion or otherwise, especially if there is any doubt about a neurological, pulmonary, cardiovascular or opthalmic disorder.*

* Warning reprinted from *The Gravity Guiding System Six Posture Program,* Gravity Guidance, Inc., 1982.

Inverted Oscillation

This exercise is excellent for the rhythmic mobilization and decompression of the joints and spinal column and the rhythmic stretching of the supporting musculature.

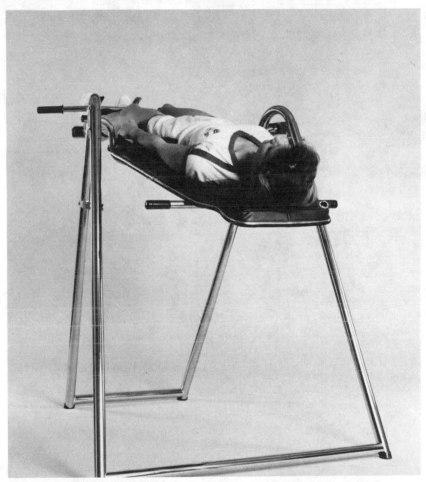

(1) Refer to the instructions supplied by the manufacturer of your system and follow them carefully. Mount your system and begin from the neutral-balance position.

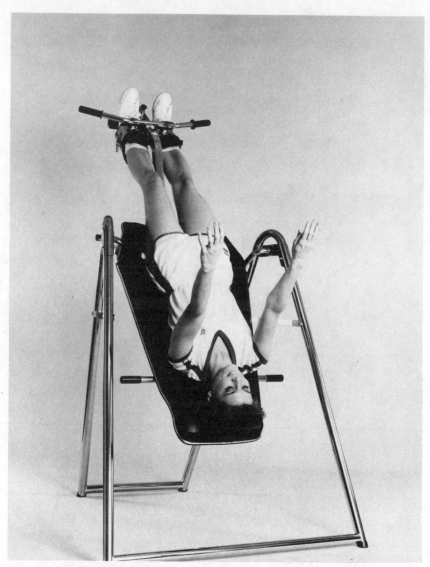

(2) Elevating your arms will change the dynamic balance of the system and begin your oscillation downward. The speed of your arm swing will determine the speed of the unit's oscillation.

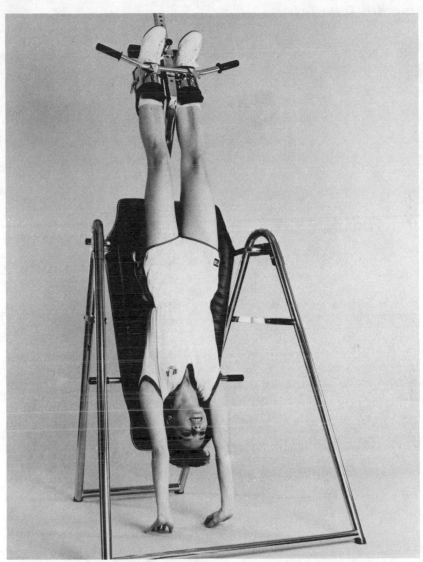

(3) Swing to the vertical position *only;* do not let your unit lock into place. Bringing your arms forward toward your torso will begin the return oscillation. Keep your rhythm slow and steady.

117

Inverted Torso Twists

This twist works the torso and back musculature. We find it is also effective in relaxing the spinal column.

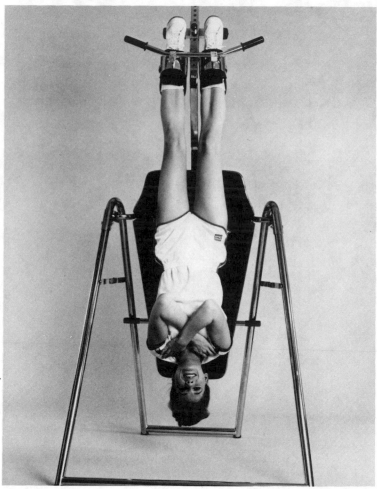

(1) Begin the exercise with your system's bed locked into the vertical position. Your arms may be crossed over your chest or hung below your head.

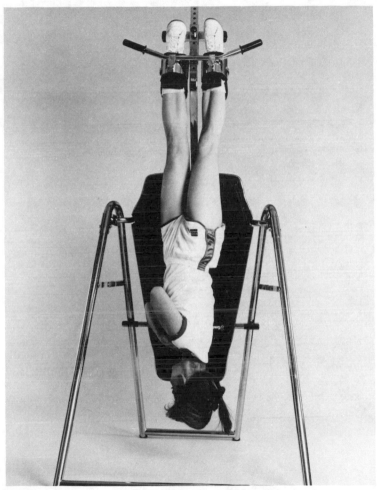

(2) Leading with your shoulder, rotate your torso to one side. Hold this position for two seconds, then return to your starting position. Rotate to the opposite side. Two rotations, one to each side, is one repetition of the exercise.

Inverted Sit-ups

In addition to working the abdominal muscles, this sit-up provides an excellent stretch for the hamstrings.

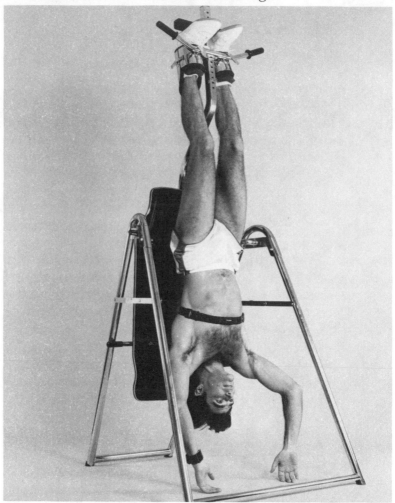

(1) Begin the exercise with the bed locked into the vertical position. Your arms should be hanging below your head.

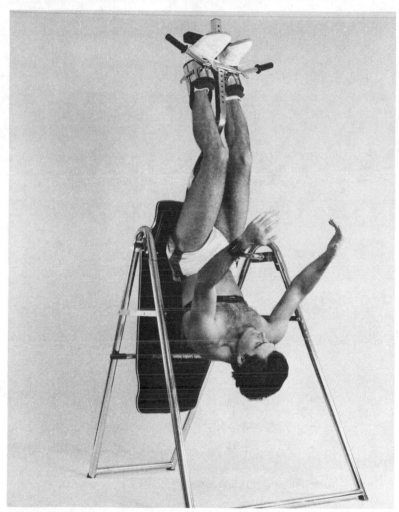

(2) Keeping your knees bent, reach up with your arms and begin to curl your torso forward, vertebrae by vertebrae. Keep your chin tucked into your chest.

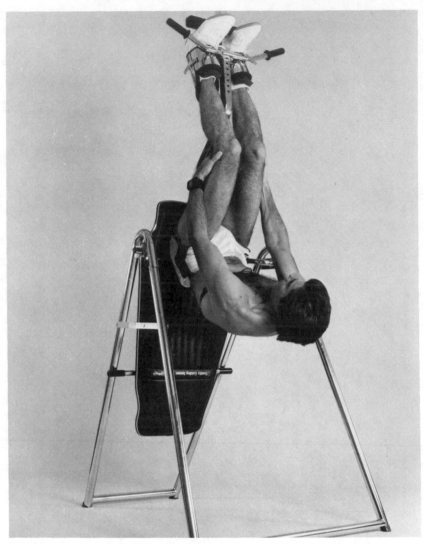

(3) Reach forward and grasp your knees as you continue to curl your torso upward.

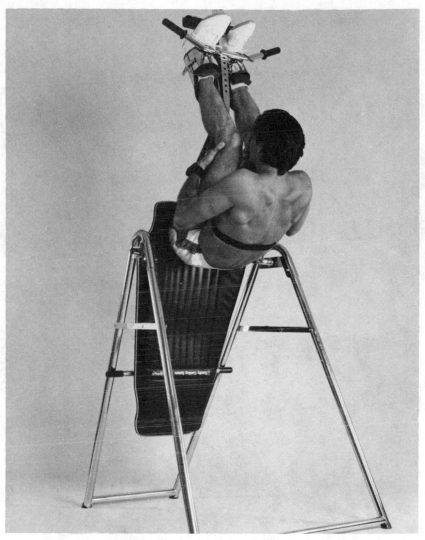

(4) Continue curling forward until your head reaches your knees, which should still be flexed. Hold this position for three seconds, then return slowly to your starting position.

Variation: Try to straighten your knees when in the sitting position.

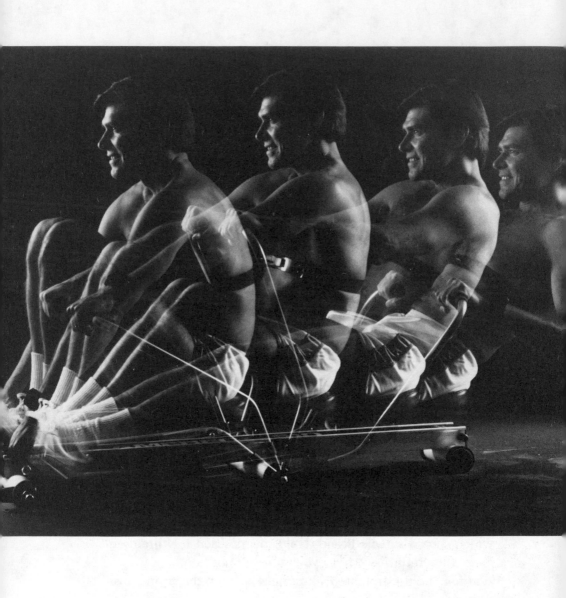

Rhythmic Endurance: Having It All

Want to develop long-term cardiovascular endurance, muscular endurance and strength simultaneously, yet avoid overload and overuse injuries, boredom, mental fatigue and exercise addiction? We've got the answer: our second access code, rhythmic endurance.

You're going to take yourself far beyond the mind-crunching, bone-jarring, thousand-step-per-mile distance runs. Using the latest in exercise science and technology, and giving a rhythmic twist to an old intensive training strategy, we can offer all of the benefits of exercise without the risks. We're going to:

- revive two old-as-the-hills but absolutely superb exercises that do it all
- introduce plyometrics, a new class of exercise used by elite athletes worldwide
- show you how to double the gains from running, cycling, rowing and the other standbys with one four-letter word: rest.

What makes it all work is rhythm, feedback and rest. The weakness of standard endurance exercise has been the inflexible adherence to continuous, long, slow distance training and "time spent" in target heart-rate zone. If five miles is good, then ten miles must be better. If twenty minutes should be spent in the zone, then thirty minutes must be better and sixty minutes must be the living end. It seems as if that old Republican campaign slogan about "a chicken in every pot" (later amended to include "two cars in every garage") must now include "and a marathon under every belt." We don't deny the aerobic and metabolic benefits of long, slow distance exercise, but how high are the costs? And why suffer if pulse-monitored rhythmic exercise can do a better job with less risk of injury?

We call our preference Rhythmic Interval Training Exercise, or RITE. It's based on the old technique of interval training, in which intervals of exercise and rest are alternated to allow the body to recover between exertions. For example, a typical interval-training run might be eight four-hundred-meter sprints with two minutes of rest between each. These brief recovery periods are actually far more than static rest; researchers have shown conclusively that true long-term physiological adaptation occurs during these intervals. Athletes in every country on earth make interval training a key part of their program, for they know that the rest periods *between* exercise bouts:

- allow for higher performance quality during each exercise interval
- allow the body to adapt to the immediate stress of exercise, which helps prevent overload and injury;
- allow time for brief mobility/flexibility exercises *during* the workout
- stimulates long-term physical adaptation that improves performance.

All those joggers who run in place at traffic lights must have missed something. What is the harm in rest?

Doing it RITE takes interval training one step further. Your rest and exercise intervals will not be dictated by a coach or a book or even your own preconceived ideas of what your body needs. They'll be based upon *heart-rate response,* in rhythm with your body's acceptance of exercise stress and its need for rest and adaptation. You'll be able to apply RITE to nearly any exercise, structuring your workout as you go, based upon the language of the body. Pulse-monitored RITE does not permit you to go too long, too fast or too far in your exercise workouts. Pulse-monitoring will make you the architect of your own fitness program instead of the spectator.

Let's use 120 heartbeats per minute as the baseline level. Obtain a pulse manually or with a monitor. Now begin your rhythmic endurance exercise—we'll take running as an example—and run easily to a pulse rate of 125. When you reach 125, slow to a walk and continue walking until your pulse returns to 120. Resume running at this point and continue until your heart rate reaches 130, five beats higher than your first rest point. Again allow your pulse to slow to 120 beats per minute; then begin running again. Your new goal is 135 beats per minute. When you reach your target zone, continue the rhythmic procedure until your workout is concluded. One added bonus: The rest intervals will allow you to access nutrition access code three, Clear Water.

When does one stop running? One excellent bit of advice from the body is a rapid acceleration from your baseline pulse to and beyond your target pulse. As you reach the point of fatigue and overload, your rapidly climbing pulse is telling you something. Listen to it. Excessive fatigue, loss of coordination and pain are all warning signals as well. And remember, cooling down should always be gradual rather than abrupt, to give the body time to re-adapt to the post-exercise state by continuing with light exercise.

We've used RITE with all of the common forms of endurance exercise and found it highly stimulating, effective and—hold on to your seat—enjoyable. We've had excellent results with the following do-it-all exercises:

The squat: Though maligned through years of misunderstanding, the correctly performed squat stands as the most complete and effective single exercise known to man. If you will pardon a time-worn but fitting cliché, the results must be seen to be believed. It will train the hamstrings and quadriceps (strengthening the knees in the process), the powerful extensors of the hips (the gluteus group in your buttocks) and the muscles of your lower back and spinal column. Rhythmic and pulse-monitored use of all these major muscle groups will cause an unparalleled *aerobic* training effect as well. Flexibility around several key joints will be improved. And you'll be creating that stable base needed for peak performance in nearly every sport from the ready positions of the shortstop and tennis player to the pre-swing stances of the batter and golfer.

We've developed the RITE program for squats that at first requires no more than a chair and your body weight. As you progress you may find that an empty barbell bar (we use a twenty-pound bar) may be all the weight you may need at first. Adding weights should be done very slowly (we do not recommend heavy weightlifting for the average person).

The Quantum Squat

In this sequence we will be using a baseline pulse of 110. You will use your own pulse rate and set your goals accordingly.

Note: Before you begin this exercise, study the photographs and instructions carefully to establish a mental image of the correct series of movements. We recommend that you practice in front of a mirror or with a partner.

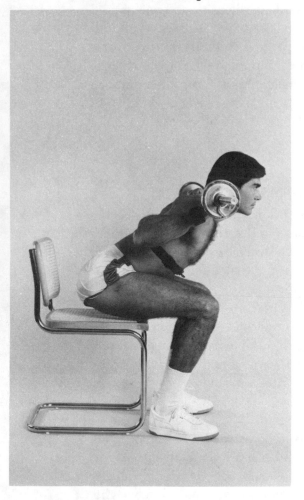

(1) Use a chair or bench of standard sitting height. Sit slightly forward on the chair, balancing the weight carefully behind your neck. Your pelvis should be in a slightly forward-tilted position; your feet should be approximately shoulder-width apart, toes pointing outward.

(2) Begin to raise yourself from the chair slowly and smoothly. At no time during the exercise should your knees extend past your toes. You can maintain this position by folding at the hip joint; your buttocks will extend backward. If you keep your ankles steady and do not allow your lower leg to swing forward, you will find this movement much easier.

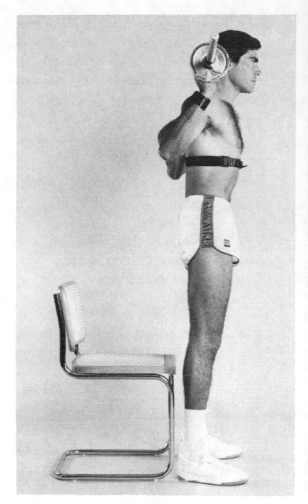

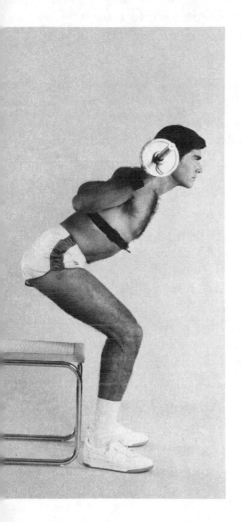

(3) Continue to straighten your torso from the hip until you are standing erect. Note that the knees are still behind the toes. Take 3 full seconds to move from the sitting position on the chair to the standing position; then take 3 seconds to return.

129

(4) Begin rhythmic sequences of 3 squats, one full deep breath, 3 squats and so on until your pulse reaches 120. Return the bar to the floor while standing and move about waiting for your pulse to drop to 110.

(5) At pulse 110, begin the same sequence until your pulse reaches 125. Stop and allow your pulse to return to 110.

(6) The same sequence is repeated at 5-beat intervals until your target pulse (for example, 145) is reached.

When do you stop? We use the same guidelines as we did with running: rapid pulse rise, fatigue, the loss of rhythm and form and the onset of pain.

This is what works for us, but by no means is it your only training strategy. As the architect, it's up to you to design the RITE program; we're only giving you the tools and setting the boundaries.

Plyometric training. Question: Where can one go to see grown men and women skipping in public? Answer: any quarter-mile track where world-class runners train. A training technique called plyometrics, which includes some drills that look for all the world like grade-school skipping, has turned the track-and-field world on its ear. Plyometrics take advantage of the elastic, rubber-band property of muscle and a system called the stretch reflex. When you perform plyometric drills, such as bounding, two phenomena occur:

- On the landing phase of a jump or a bound, the leg muscles that normally *contract* to propel you get stretched. Watch and feel the muscles of your front thigh, your quadriceps, as you squat downward; the muscles are lengthened as a rubber band might be. The energy stored in these muscles, as in a rubber band, can be used to propel you to a greater height on the next jump or bound.
- When the muscles are stretched upon landing, the nervous system employs a rapid protective system called the stretch reflex. If sensors detect that the quadriceps are being stretched, the body prevents them from being over-

stretched and torn by making them contract. This "reflex contraction" helps you jump or bound still higher, adding to the effect of the elastic rebound.

Apparently, using the elastic recoil and stretch-reflex properties of muscle during training have a great carryover to athletic performance. We are confident that plyometrics are here to stay and should play a role in nonathletic training as well.

We've included examples of plyometric bounding drills (a term you'll appreciate as you merrily bound along) in the rhythmic endurance section. Done properly, with careful attention to pulse and body talk, you'll get some surprising results. The cardiovascular training effect is expected, but the high-knee action will develop strong, resilient quadriceps and flexible hamstrings, and will make a significant contribution to your pelvic stability. We suggest that you try the high-knee walk first if you're a novice; the high-knee skip is a more advanced variation.

Stairway to heaven.
If you thought all those athletes looked silly bounding, head over to the football stadium to see the swimming, water polo, track and soccer teams running up the bleachers. Stair-running, like the squat, is one of the most completely effective exercises you can do. Talk about endurance and strength in one package: each step can be considered a one-legged squat, and as you now know, major-muscle-group activity means high aerobic quality.

We have done quite successful stair workouts at home with a single flight of steps, following a strategy much like the squat routine we described earlier. You should have the picture by now: climb until you hit a target pulse, then rest and recover by allowing your pulse to return to a lower level. Resume climbing to a five-beat-higher target, then rest and recover again. You won't even have to run the stairs at first; walking is stressful enough for novices. As your strength and endurance increase you can progress from walking from every step to every other step.

131

A final bit of advice: Most of the stress from stair-climbing comes with the descent. *Don't ever run down the stairs.* Consider the rest on the trip down part of the rhythm.

Ordering Everything on the Menu

The many values of variety and feedback are best highlighted in our menu workout. Use your rowing machine, bike, treadmill or staircase for a new twist on circuit-training. Rather than set an arbitrary time or distance for any exercise, do it RITE on one exercise, then move to the next and repeat the process from scratch. Here's the idea: Start on the treadmill, gradually warming up with pulse monitoring. Follow the same guidelines described earlier, but after reaching your target heart-rate zone, allow yourself to recover, then move to the rowing machine and begin anew. Then work rhythmically from exercise to exercise until your target zone is reached in each mode. We can't think of a more enjoyable and effective way to exercise. Continue your round-robin program until your body informs you that it's time to cool down.

The Rhythmic Endurance Program

Choose from the options listed below, or adapt a favorite form of exercise that uses the major muscle groups. Aim for variety in your daily workout sessions, with at least fifteen to twenty minutes spent in the region of your target heart-rate zone. If your body says yes, you may continue working rhythmically. Don't forget that significant inroads into your body's fat stores are not made until you've been active for at least forty-five minutes. You may combine two or more rhythmic endurance exercises within a single workout.

An added benefit of the rhythmic endurance program is the exceptional degree of strength that can be applied to your daily activities and sporting interests. Experiment with as many of these choices as possible, and remember that variety is one of the keys to both good nutrition and good exercise.

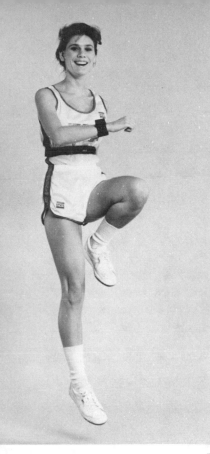

Squats
High-Knee Walk/Skip
   We recommend that you begin
with the high-knee walk, progress
to skipping and then add the
high-knee movement to the skip-
ping phase of the exercise.
Stair-Climbing
Hill-Climbing
Running (outdoors or on a tread-
mill)
Skipping

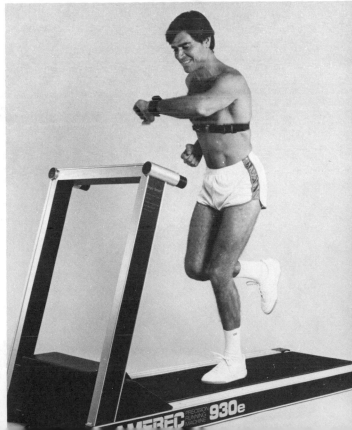

Mini-Trampolining

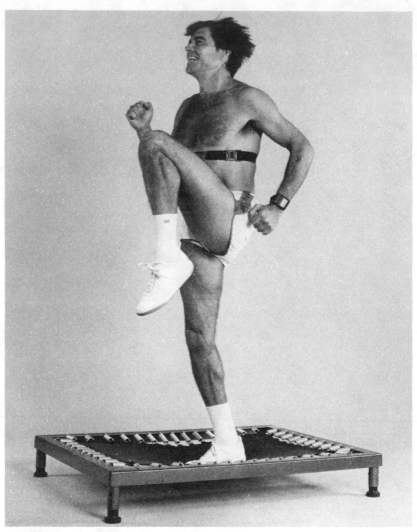

This is an inexpensive and effective choice of rhythmic endurance training. The high knee exercise shown is one of several ways to develop endurance, strength and pelvic balance simultaneously.

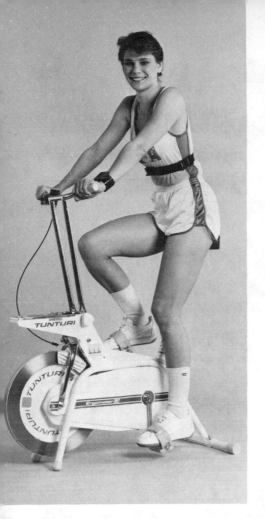

Cycling

Cycling can be done indoors or outdoors. Indoor cycling is a low stress yet effective exercise. The use of bicycle ergometers like this one allows accurate measurement of workload and pedalling speed, information that can be used in designing your workout.

Rowing
Indoor rowing machines are booming in popularity and with good reason. Few muscles escape this whole body workout.
Swimming
Jumping Rope
Cross-country Skiing
Roller and Ice Skating

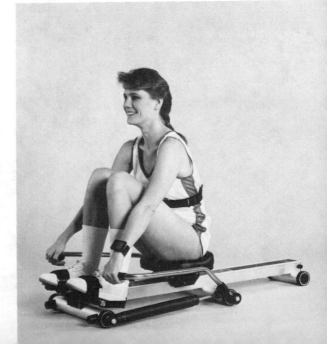

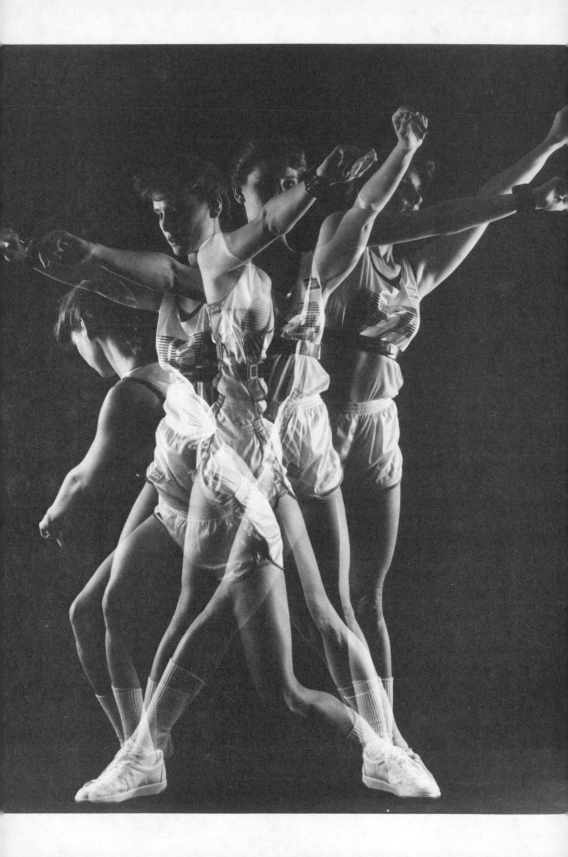

Multi-Joint Patterning Exercise: The Final Code

As you must realize by now, we're big believers in synergism, that mysterious but achievable state in which the whole exceeds the sum of the parts. We're convinced that the body is synergistic and that one of the secrets to high performance is multiple-joint rather than isolation training. There *are* times when one would want to focus on, or isolate, a particular muscle; rehabilitation and bodybuilding are two examples. But that's *not* how the body performs. In fact, some fascinating research recently compared the muscles and the motor control systems of concert pianists, elite Olympic swimmers and weight lifters with those of normal, healthy adults. The investigators concluded that it was in *orchestrating the work of several muscles, not in the control of individual muscles,* that the elite performers excelled.

Given then that (1) the body works in three dimensions with multiple joints (wrist plus elbow plus shoulder, or ankle plus knee plus hip, for example), and that (2) Olympic-level performances result from the efficient coordination of multiple joints and muscles, we have made multijoint exercise our third and final exercise access code. Multijoint patterning exercises are performed repetitively, smoothly and in patterns so that you learn to move with proper coordination. The exercises we have included are but a small fraction of those possible, and should provide you with both a place to start and a baseline for future evaluation. For fitness and optimal athletic performance, look for those exercises that teach the body to coordinate its parts into movement patterns, not isolate them.

Finally, many multijoint exercises do triple duty: they serve as multijoint-patterns, rhythmic-endurance and pelvic-balance exercises; the squat and high-knee skipping are perfect examples. If you select a multijoint exercise that can be pulse-monitored for rhythmic endurance purposes, you're catching on.

137

The MultiJoint Exercise Sampler

Wall Push-ups

This is the easiest of the four push-up variations you'll find here, and the one we recommend for beginners. Like all push-ups, it develops the muscles of the chest, shoulders and upper and lower arms.

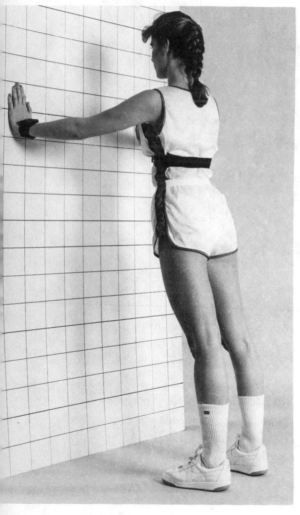

(1) Stand a foot or so away from the wall. Place your arms six to twelve inches beyond your shoulder width on either side. Keep your abdomen contracted.

(2) Lean into the wall, keeping your body in a straight line from shoulder to heel. If you keep your elbows extended to the sides, you will be working the pectoral muscles of your chest; if they are along your sides, you will be working your triceps. Keep your abdominals contracted. Your heels may rise off the floor, but this indicates poor hamstring/calf flexibility. Return to your starting position.

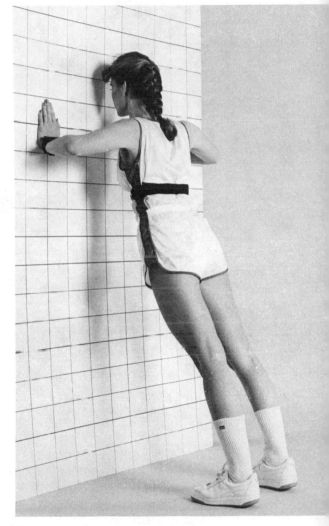

Chair Push-ups

A somewhat more difficult version of wall push-ups.

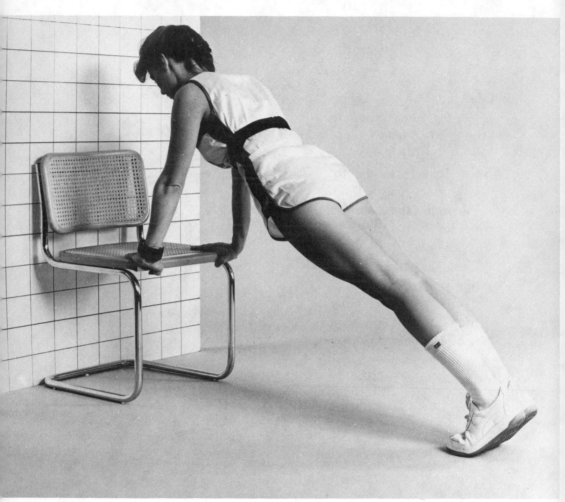

(1) Place your arms on either side of the chair. Keeping your arms straight, walk your legs out until you achieve the position shown in the photograph.

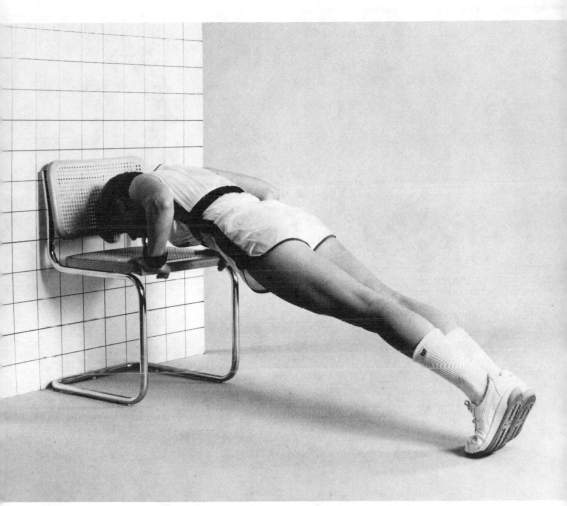

(2) Lower yourself slowly to the chair. The position of the elbows shown in the photograph allows both the triceps and pectoral muscles to share the load. Raise yourself slowly, still keeping your body in a straight line.

Floor Push-ups

The classic. Need we say more?

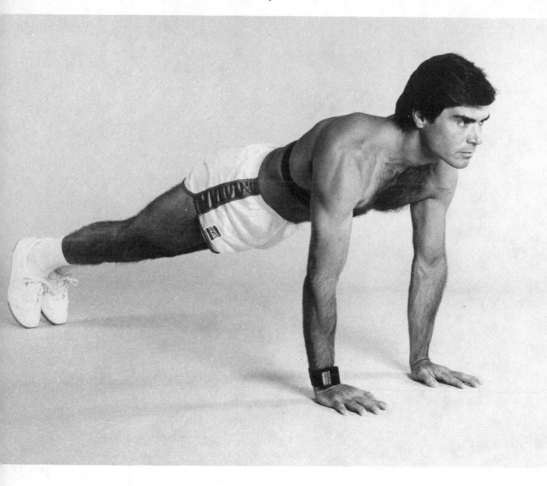

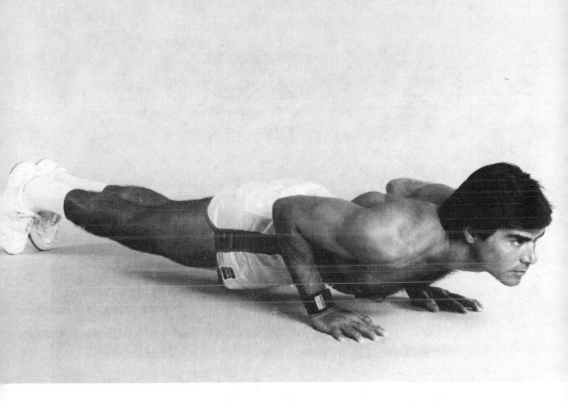

You may further increase the difficulty of this exercise by doing these push-ups on closed fists or on your fingertips. Here the elbows are shown in the triceps-emphasized position.

Inverted Chair Push-ups

This is the most difficult version of the push-up for the advanced athlete.

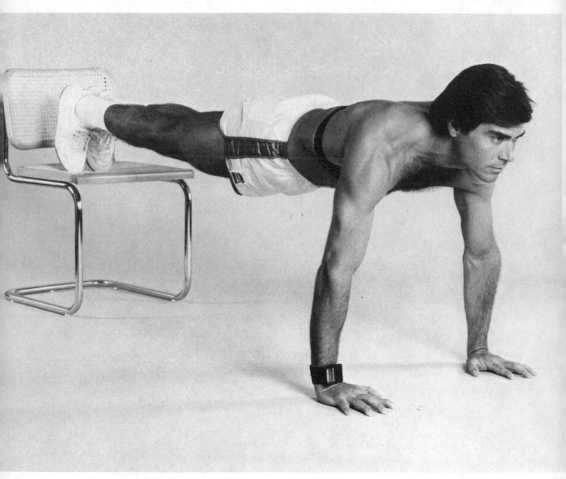

(1) This push-up follows the same basic formula as the preceding variations. The difficulty of the exercise increases the more your feet are raised.

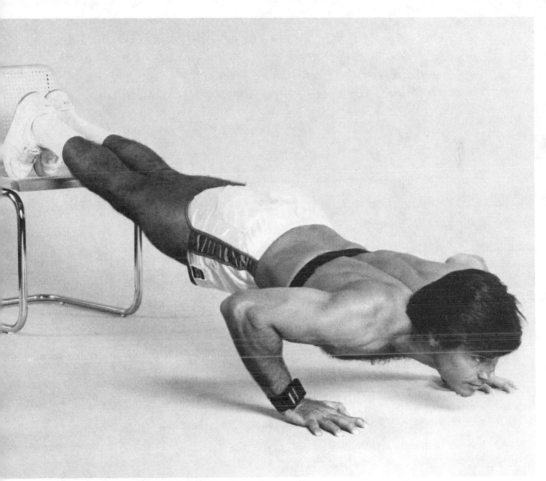

(2) Note how the body is held in a straight line.

Modified Barbell Curl

This variation on the classic weight-lifting exercise offers greater development of the upper arms and shoulders with decreased stress on the elbow joints. We suggest practicing this exercise without a bar to get used to the range of motion.

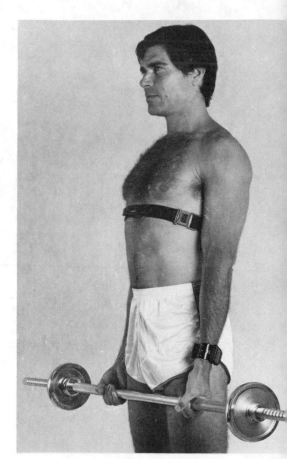

(1) Stand erect with your feet comfortably apart. Your abdominal and thigh muscles should be contracted. Hold the bar with your hands just outside your thighs.

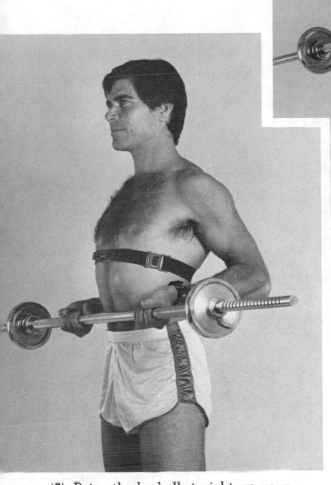

(2) Bring the barbell straight up your body, following a vertical path. This will be easier to accomplish if you feel your elbows moving up and back. Your wrists should be in the slightly downward extension as shown. Try to minimize any arching of your back; you might try tilting your pelvis forward slightly.

(3) Now swing your elbows forward and curl your wrists toward your shoulders. In this way the biceps are still the main muscle responsible for the movement, but most of the stress has been taken off of the elbow joints. Slowly return to your starting position.

147

Chin-ups

This is still one of the best multi-joint choices, working the muscles of the chest, shoulder, upper and lower arms.

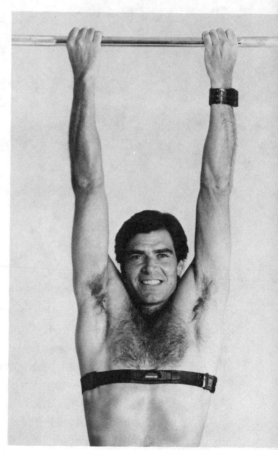

(1) Grasp the bar just outside or in line with your shoulders.

148

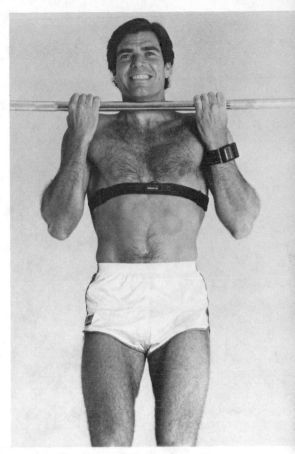

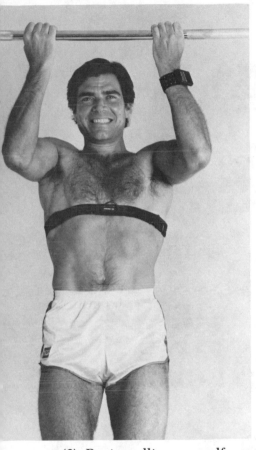

(3) Continue pulling yourself upward until your chin "rests" on top of the bar. Hold this position for a count of two. Lower yourself slowly and smoothly. Do not drop into the starting position; work downward to a count of five to ten seconds for maximum training gains.

(2) Begin pulling yourself upward, keeping your abdomen contracted. Try not to arch your back too much; a moderate forward pelvic tilt will help.

Modified French Curl

This variation of the curl exercise reduces stress on the elbow while doubling the number of working muscles.

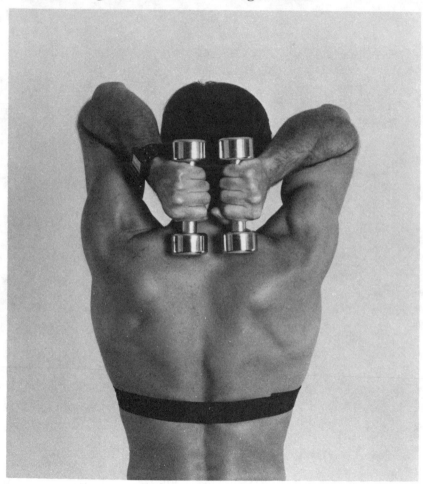

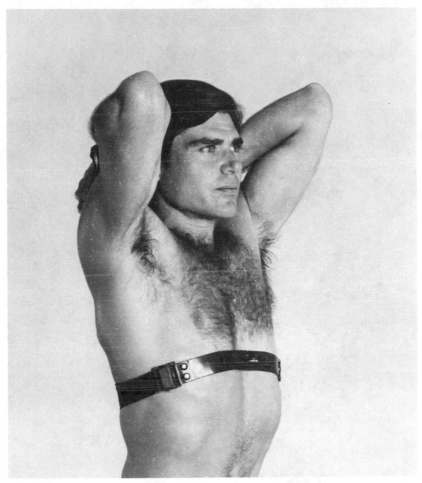

(1) Grasp a dumbbell in each hand with your palms facing upward; bring your arms behind your head. Your palms should now be facing forward; your elbows are held high and outward at a slight angle. Minimize any arching of your back by contracting your abdominal muscles.

151

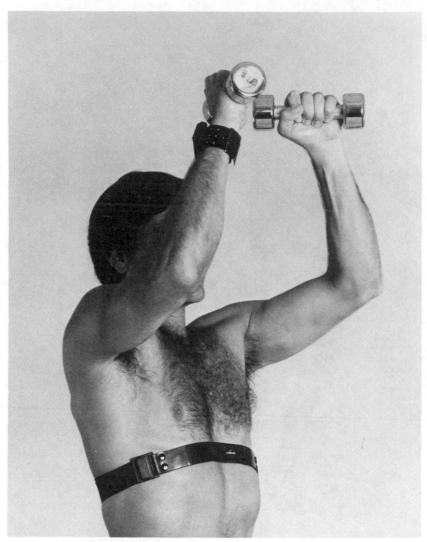

(2) Extend your forearms, rotating your hands outward. Your elbows may drop slightly.

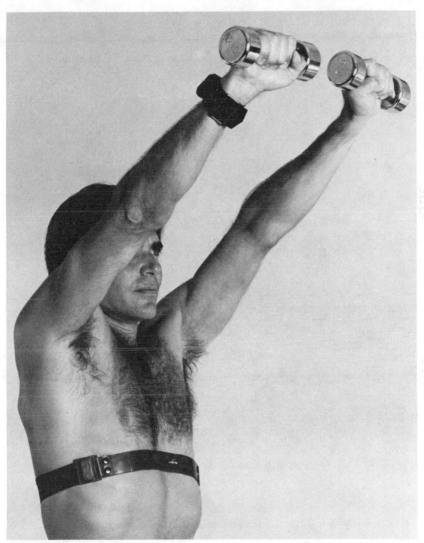

(3) Continue extending your forearms; your hands should be fully rotated; your palms should be facing downward. Reverse your movements and return to your starting position.

Discus Throw

This mobility exercise takes nearly every joint and muscle through a good range of motion. It is an excellent contributor to pelvic balance as it stretches the iliopsoas group of muscles, which are frequently the cause of back pain.

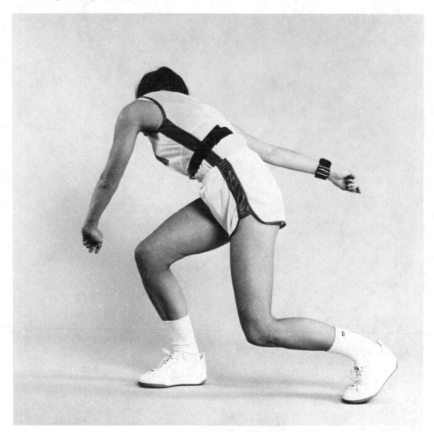

(1) Stand erect with your feet comfortably apart. Step forward, putting your weight on your front leg. Twist your torso down and around as far as it is comfortable for you to do so, bending your knees deeply. Bring one arm back as if you are preparing to throw a discus.

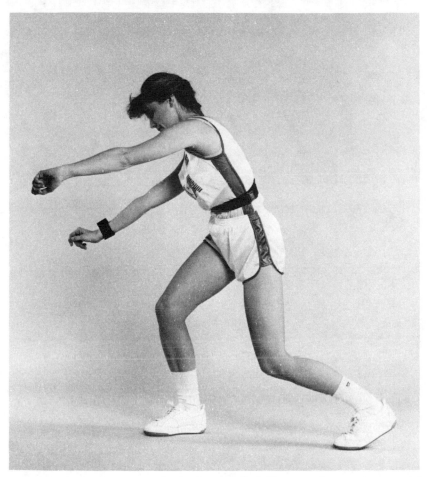

(2) Begin to rotate your body forward, following the movement of your torso with both arms.

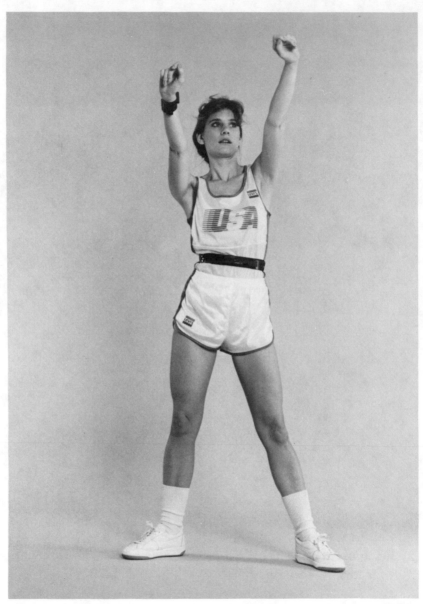

(3) Continue rotating your body forward, preparing to "release the discus."

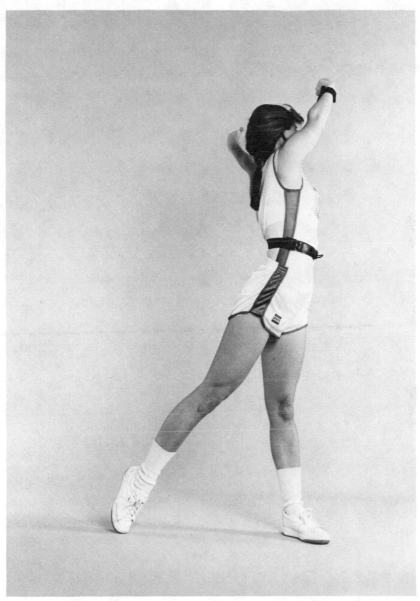

(4) Follow through on the throw, twisting your torso so that it gets a good stretch. Return to your starting position and repeat on the opposite side.

157

Standing Buttock Kick

An effective mobility exercise for the muscles in the front and back thigh.

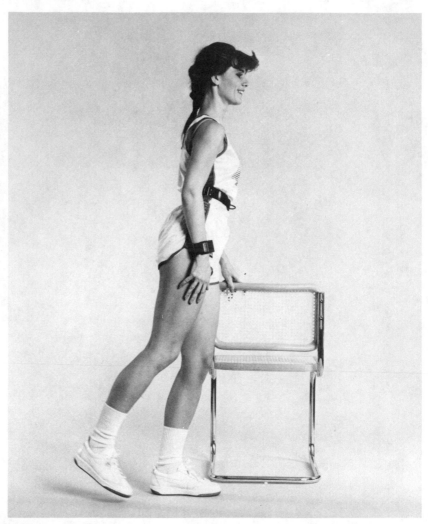

(1) Stand tall, with your hand resting on the back of a chair or a ballet bar for balance. Begin the movement with a slight backward swing of your outside leg.

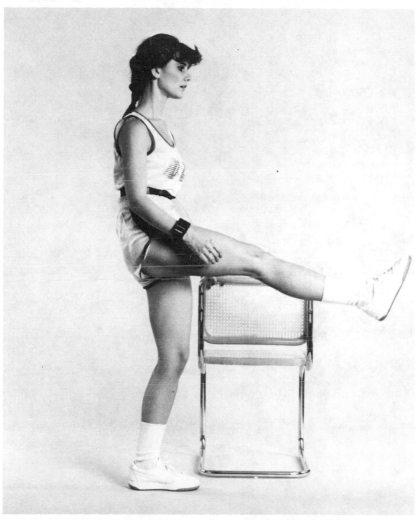

(2) Swing the leg forward to a comfortable height.

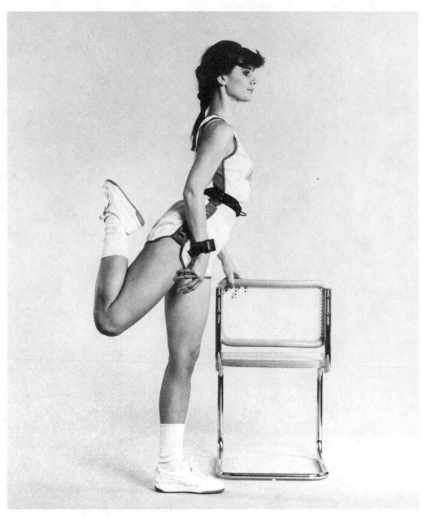

(3) Swing the leg backward, flexing your knee and bringing your foot toward your buttocks. Return to your starting position.

160

Running Buttock Kick

This movement can be used while running to improve the flexibility of the quadriceps, the muscle in the front of the thigh.

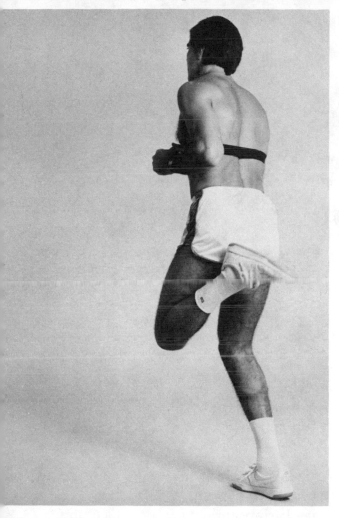

Leg Swing

This is an excellent exercise for developing the mobility of the hip joint and inner and outer thigh muscles.

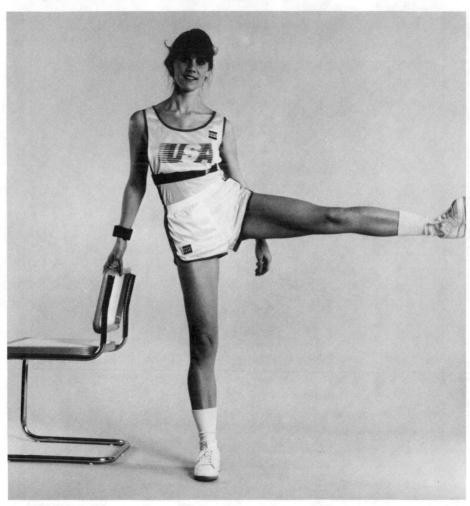

(1) Stand erect, with your hand resting on the back of a chair for balance. Swing your outside leg to the side as high as you can without discomfort. Extend the leg fully.

162

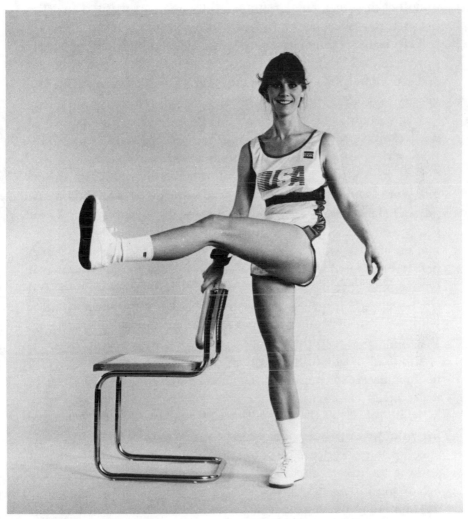

(2) Swing the leg across your body, gently stretching your outer thigh. You may flex your knee slightly to allow a greater range of motion. Return to the starting position.

Putting the Codes Together: Quantum Workouts

If we've done our job and convinced you that *you* can be the architect of your fitness program, you won't be surprised that the next ten pages are not crammed with Quantum workouts.

The means to our Quantum exercise goals—health, peak performance and longevity—are provided by the three access codes and attention to the principles creating dynamic balance: rhythm, variety and adaptation.

What would we do if we really had our way? In an ideal world we'd exercise several times a day, just as we would eat several times a day. Small doses of both food *and* exercise are more easily digestible, and the several-hour-long metabolic boost from exercise would end up lasting all day. We'd start each day with a few pelvic-balance exercises (but only because *our* bodies are ready for it at seven A.M.; yours may prefer to wait, and that's fine). Rhythmic endurance work would follow, about thirty minutes' worth before breakfast. At lunch we'd go for a brisk walk and crown it with some fiber-based carbohydrates, lean-source protein and clear water. (Clever how we worked in that synergy, no?) After work we'd head home for some additional multijoint exercising. We might even cap the day with a relaxing walk after dinner.

You don't reside in this ideal world, of course, so you'll have to be imaginative in your use of the access codes. If your body likes to wake up around ten A.M. but you're at work at eight-thirty, a morning run is not the wisest choice. See if you can fit in an easy five minutes of pelvic balance work and save the rhythmic endurance for later. Perhaps you *can* try the old but invaluable trick of parking the car at the far end of the lot at work or getting off the bus or subway a stop early.

Too busy at lunch for a walk? You only have time to eat at your desk? Perhaps you can sneak in a free ten or fifteen minutes during slack late-morning or mid-afternoon hours. A walk might be just the thing to perk you up and burn a few calories.

One option you won't want to take is the get-it-all-done-on-the-weekend trick. There is no surer path to overuse injury than cramming all your exercise needs into one massive workout. Search each day for the time to insert pelvic balance work, or ten or fifteen minutes of rhythmic endurance, or multijoint patterning. The Quantum You *knows* the time is there if you want it to be.

The following three steps provide the basis of your participation in the Quantum Exercise program.

Step I

Select a variety of exercises from the Quantum Exercise codes:

- Pelvic Balance
- Rhythmic Endurance
- Multijoint Patterning.

Choose your main "events" (such as a running-based program or a cycling-based program) according to your own preference and requirements. A variety of exercises built around your "main event" will assure a well-rounded program.

Step II

Apply the Quantum principle of rhythm. The frequency, intensity and duration of exercise training will be determined by tapping into your body's rhythms—for example, your pulse rate.

Step III

Use personally constructed simulation cycles to direct and reinforce positive changes in your program and yourself. Follow the signals provided by your body and mind; then feedback to adjust and redirect your program accordingly.

As in nutrition, a dynamically balanced program based on the exercise codes will set off a chemical chain reaction resulting in physiological, structural and psychological benefits. The ball is now in your court. It's time for *you* to call the plays.

You've put yourself in the center of the arena. You've got the force of mind for it. You've got the energy source and you've got the delivery system. The next step is the big leap.

THE QUANTUM LEAP

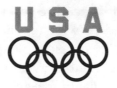

T HE VOICE is as vivid in our ears today as it was during that television and radio broadcast in 1962. He made the impossible sound so possible.

"Why, some say, the moon? Why choose this as our goal? And, they may well ask, why climb the highest mountain? Why, thirty-five years ago, fly the Atlantic? Why does Rice play Texas? We choose to go to the moon!"

That was John F. Kennedy's impossible dream in 1962. In every crowd there is always one individual who believes and who can lead others to believe. Seven years after Kennedy's preposterous declaration of intent, we were witness to another television and radio broadcast that made history:

"I'm going to step off the ramp now. That's one small step for man, and one giant leap for mankind!" The *Eagle* had landed.

167

After the quarter-million-mile return trip to earth, Neil Armstrong was interviewed on his reactions to having become the first human being to set foot on the moon. In addition to sharing his joy, awe and pride in being part of an elite team with unity of purpose, Armstrong also provided us with insight into his own depth of character when he said: "Ever since I was a little boy, I dreamed I would do something important in aviation."

Dare *we* dream of a Quantum leap? Is it foolish to imagine being the first woman president? Indira Gandhi and Golda Meir didn't think so. What was Margaret Thatcher thinking of when she—at age twenty-one, still living over her father's grocery store—had the audacity to see herself as prime minister of England? And what about Helen Keller, who, though blind and deaf, dedicated her life to helping the less fortunate? How dare Wilma Rudolph take the brace off her polio-withered leg and seven years later win three gold medals as the fastest woman in the world at the Rome Olympic Games? The Quantum leap belongs to the believers who dare to be different!

There is a tribe of South American Indians whose members have been dying prematurely of a mysterious disease for many generations. It was finally discovered that the malady was caused by the bite of an insect that lives in the walls of their adobe mud dwellings. The Indians have several possible solutions: They can destroy their infested homes and rebuild them with new adobe blocks that have been chemically treated; they can destroy the insects in their homes with an insecticide; they can migrate to another area where there are no such insects; or they can continue to live and die young, just as they have done for generations. Ironically, they have chosen to stay just as they are and accept their fate.

Many individuals have a similar attitude about personal development and fitness. They can see the possibilities for others, but they can't imagine it happening to themselves.

As you grasp the Quantum Fitness principles and build your own program toward greater excellence, there will be many who will try to rain on your parade. Always remember that misery loves company and that most of your fair-weather peers would just as soon you stay out of shape with them at their level rather than see you move up and out. That's why there is so much resistance to an innovative idea or concept. New ideas require change. Change requires risk and effort.

WELCOME TO THE FIVE-PERCENT CLUB

In his syndicated radio program *Our Changing World,* our friend Earl Nightingale, who many consider to be the dean of American motivators, observes that from our earliest history there have always been two main groups of people. One group is large, consisting of about 95 percent of any society. The other is small, about five percent. It is uncanny how populations seem to insist on splitting into these two groups: the large group of followers and the small group of leaders. For example, out of all the young individuals who start at the same level at age twenty-five, only 5 percent are financially secure by the time they are sixty-five. They didn't necessarily come from better families, or grow up on the right side of the railroad tracks, or even attend the finest universities; they simply played the game of life to win. Barring a catastrophe any individual can save enough money during a forty-year career to be financially secure at sixty-five. But only 5 percent make the effort to learn enough early in the game to set goals and save before it is too late.

Every city has a public library crammed full of knowledge that is absolutely free if you get the books back on time. But can you guess how many individuals continue to learn and develop their minds after they get out of high school or college? You're right— about 5 percent!

The reason more individuals don't step out from the 95 percent and stay involved in a lifelong development program is the fear of alienation from their peers. The greatest driving force of human nature after meeting physical needs is the craving to be appreciated. And the opposite of being appreciated is to feel left out of the group. The fear of rejection, or being out of step with your peers, progresses into the fear of change, which includes the fear of charting unknown waters, of being first and of sacrificing external security. The fear of change becomes the fear of success, which is manifested in guilt associated with our natural desire for excellence and self-gratification. The fear of change and the fear of success are the negative currents that stun the 95 percent in their lower orbits and cause them to gravitate into a sedentary life of conformity and bad habits.

As they get older the 95 percent make decisions that narrow their opportunities and alternatives for personal growth. They select only a few friends out of the thousands they meet, usually people with whom they agree, thus limiting their exposure to fresh ideas. They choose a static educational level, which in turn determines to a great extent their jobs and associates. They eat the same foods by force of habit—usually foods that are not good for them. They are consistent in their lack of physical exercise and personal grooming. From day to day, comfortable in their safe, established ways, their bodies rust out rather than wear out.

You have looked at the shackles the 95 percent have placed upon themselves by apathy, and in a moment of truth you have made a declaration of independence. You see being different as having higher personal and professional standards of excellence. You see being different as synonymous with striving for higher performance, better health and a longer, more productive life. You see being different as putting more time, thought and effort into all that you do. You see being different as taking the calculated risk, knowing that you will create your future security by plans and actions that will set you free—and make you able to stand apart.

You are different because you dare to consider the existence of a Quantum leap in your own fitness universe. You are different because you have chosen to use facts instead of fads for your mental, nutritional and exercise principles. But mostly you are different because you dare to separate yourself from the pack and place yourself at center stage. You have chosen to participate, rather than observe. And this, as we have learned from Quantum physics, will dramatically change the outcome of your life.

THE WHOLE IS GREATER THAN THE SUM OF ITS PARTS

As you participate in building your own Quantum Fitness program, take heart! At first you'll be a bit skeptical and unsure. You'll feel like an amateur in what seems to be in a professional's lofty domain. There will be myths to discard and new concepts to understand and embrace. There will be new techniques and routines to learn—new habits to be formed in place of the old ones. Your first unsteady steps forward will become rhythmic strides. And, almost without noticing, you'll break away from one energy and performance level and move toward the level of excellence. You won't be able to pinpoint it in your fitness diary. You won't monitor it on your bathroom scale. It won't be measured in miles, pounds, inches or minutes. After the first few weeks of little steps, you'll suddenly discover that you have taken that special leap. And you won't remember the transition from one place to the other.

Let's sum up the important elements of the Quantum Fitness program and review the simplicity and harmony with which they connect to give you the breakthrough to personal excellence.

First, there are the three Quantum principles—*adaptation, variety* and *rhythm*—which will work to bring your personal universe into a state of dynamic balance. The universe within you is sensitive to the exact form in which the fundamental laws of physics manifest themselves. Since nature's orchestration is always changing, you are constantly adapting to your changing environment by monitoring feedback and responding to your unique, internal rhythms. Your open, inquiring mind, combined with your new nutrition and exercise habits—rich in their variety—are your means to this dynamic balance.

171

Next, there are the five Olympic rings, which are the connecting links in your fitness arena:

Ring One You make the difference. You are the maestro of your Quantum Fitness symphony. You do not fit into someone else's fitness program; you design your own.

Ring Two Your mind is the Quantum Force. It is mind over menus and mind over muscles. Your mind is what matters in Quantum Fitness.

Ring Three There are no miracle diets. Olympic athletes, just like you, must draw upon a balanced variety of foods, providing nutrients in multiple combinations to fuel their biofires for Quantum Nutrition.

Ring Four Physical exertion and recovery using feedback-controlled rhythm are central concepts in Quantum Exercise. It is knowing how the muscles and joints move together, and listening to your body talk, that makes the Quantum Exercise program work.

Ring Five The *connection* of the five rings, and their wonderful interdependence, set off the chain reaction: a Quantum Fitness leap.

Remember the connections? They are the eight simple access codes that enable you to break through the fitness maze and unlock the door to your true potential.

The first two were the mental Quantum access codes of *adaptive relaxation* and *simulation cycles.* Using adaptive relaxation techniques, you learned how to manage stress and make your mind more receptive to new input. Using the simulation cycles of feedforward self-talk and feedback self-talk, you developed the skill to construct visual, verbal and emotional previews of coming attractions, which locked in new life-style, nutritional and exercise attitudes.

172

Armed with a deeper understanding of the power of the Quantum Force in your mind, you integrated the three nutrition Quantum access codes of *fiber-based carbohydrates, lean-source proteins* and *clear water.* Applying these simple access codes to a new wider variety of foods, you set off a cascade of positive effects from your daily energy input.

The final three Quantum access codes were *pelvic balance,* which became the foundation for all purposeful and healthful movement; *rhythmic endurance,* which became the means to maximize cardiovascular and muscular adaptation while minimizing the possibility of overload, injury and disease; and *multijoint patterning exercise,* which set the boundaries within which training can enhance the brain's ability to coordinate its wondrously complex system of bones and muscles.

The three Quantum principles, blending with the eight simple Quantum access codes, were refined into a basic definition of what the Quantum Fitness program really means. It is your handle to grasp and your baton to carry as you put it all together into your leap forward. What *is* Quantum Fitness? *It is the dynamically balanced organization of your exercise and nutrition programs and your mind that uses simple access codes to unlock your hidden potential and achieve health, performance and longevity.*

Will Quantum Fitness work for you? We believe it will. Using just the mental part of the Quantum plan, you can become more self-directed and take more personal responsibility for the outcome of your life. You can raise your self-image, which in turn will automatically raise your level of preparation and expectation for your performance. You can learn to relax and respond more effectively to the stresses in your life. You can learn to control your eating habits and improve your health and your appearance. Instead of fasting and gorging, you can combine planning and variety. You can master the technique of visualizing yourself as you would like to be, and see yourself as more playful, energetic and alive.

Using only the nutritional part of the Quantum plan, you can improve the amount and quality of fuel you take into that marvelous space-vehicle you call your body, your one and only transportation system for life. You can help prevent diabetes, hypertension, coronary and artery problems, certain kinds of cancer and other dietary problems. You can learn to eat for energy and enjoyment, not out of frustration, boredom or compensation.

Using only the exercise part of the Quantum plan, you can increase the strength of your muscles and the flexibility of your muscles and joints. You can maximize your physical performance both in terms of immediate power and endurance. Through proper exercise, over time you can improve your physical appearance and, most important, minimize the risk of cardiovascular and other stress- or sedentary–life-style–related diseases.

But when you apply Quantum Fitness as a whole system, the result is greater than the sum of the individual parts. Your nutrition program will work because of your mental attitude, and you will discover new energy and motivation for high performance. Your exercise program will actually decrease your desire for improper amounts and types of foods. Your physical activity will have a positive effect on your mental attitude, and you will become more optimistic and more excited about your goals. Your mind will function better because it thinks better, is fueled better and benefits from your body's exercise. And this new vitality will spark your mind to greater challenges, which in turn will accelerate your body into new, productive activities and orbits. The impossible will become possible, then real.

Does this Quantum leap really occur? Can this really happen to you?

Think back to Lake Placid, New York. It is the winter of 1980. They were an unlikely group. There were twenty of them, averaging twenty-two years of age. Just a collection of young intelligent guys who were willing to channel their egos, and subject themselves to a demanding training program.

According to Herb Brooks, their coach, he wanted adaptable in-

174

dividuals who could think faster and skate better than their opponents. "The ignorant people, the self-centered people, the people who don't want to expand their thoughts—they're not going to be the real good athletes," Brooks said in an interview. He used a special psychological test to select his final team. Rather than trying to assemble superstars, he was seeking team players, who could respond to stress and seize the moment under pressure.

It was an impossible, almost ludicrous assignment. The Russians had always been in a class by themselves, with everybody else in a distant second class. Brooks sought the counsel of other coaches who had successfully trained world-class athletes and learned everything he could about power, endurance, flexibility, nutrition, loading, recovery time, pulse rates and peak points. And because his players were resilient enough and eager enough to learn, he was able to make strides. They were willing to dare to try.

The US team was ranked number seven in an eight-team field and had the toughest schedule in the tournament, facing the Swedes and Czechs, ranked second and third in the world. To make matters worse, the Americans had been blown off the ice by the Russians in the final exhibition game by a score of 10 to 3 at Madison Square Garden just prior to the 1980 Winter Games at Lake Placid. Good luck on coming in fourth!

What happened? Was it because they were so young and inexperienced that they didn't believe that they couldn't achieve their goals? Didn't they watch the evening news enough or read the morning paper enough to become discouraged? Was it because they were still unspoiled and uncynical? Was their weakness of inexperience actually their greatest strength?

We think it was more. We believe they broke through and experienced a Quantum leap. Down their competitors went—first Sweden, then Norway, next Czechoslovakia, then Rumania, even West Germany—always under a burst in the third period. How could the American team come from behind like that? How dare they?

Then the impossible happened. Before the game Brooks had

175

told them that this was their moment in history. That it was going to happen. Ten minutes to go. US 4, USSR 3. The crowd fell silent. And then it *was* history. The horn blew and there was the bedlam of victory, the sprawling, leaping, hugging, crying. The pandemonium and the hurling of hockey sticks. The red-white-and-blue flags. The realization of triumph.

As individuals they were good. As a team they were a transcendental winning machine, a troop of unknown kids who became the best ice hockey team in the world. They captured the heart of a nation hungry for any morsel of international pride. They had been totally committed to their dream and in the process had reflected what all of us had always yearned to see in ourselves. That the whole can be greater than the sum of its parts. That mind and body can be melded to make the impossible real.

DARING TO BE GREAT

What Herb Brooks's and Earl Nightingale's 5 percent always knew was that the power of the mind, applied through the miracle of the human body, can do anything. Quantum Fitness is the framework to which you will apply that power. It is for the 95 percent *and* the five percent, the nonathlete as well as the Olympic medalist.

The deck is stacked in your favor; the chain reactions are waiting to be set off. You have five separate Olympic rings in your hands. Link them and let their synergy change your life.

Think of your life as a marvelous jigsaw puzzle. It is the structure, the interdependence—the *fit*—of the pieces that makes the whole rings work. Like Rembrandt's colors and Shakespeare's words, you can create an enduring masterpiece. We've made the Quantum leap to personal excellence possible. It's up to *you* to make it real.

BIBLIOGRAPHY

Here is a list of books we personally recommend for further reading.

Yalouris, Nicolaos. *The Eternal Olympics.* New Rochelle, NY: Caratzas Brothers, 1979. We recommend this book as an excellent overview of the history of the Olympics.

Readings on Quantum Physics, Science and Philosophy

Ayensu, Edward S. *The Rhythms of Life.* New York: Crown, 1981.

Bohm, David. *Wholeness and the Implicate Order.* London: Routledge and Kegan Paul, 1980.

Bronowski, Jacob. *Science and Human Values.* New York: Harper & Row, 1965.

Capra, Fritjof. *The Tao of Physics.* New York: Bantam, 1977.

Pagels, Heinz R. *The Cosmic Code: Quantum Physics as the Law of Nature.* New York: Simon & Schuster, 1982.

Prigogine, Ilya. *From Being to Becoming.* San Francisco: W. H. Freeman, 1980.

Schrodinger, Erwin. *What Is Life?* New York: Cambridge University Press, 1944.

Wolf, Fred Alan. *Taking the Quantum Leap.* San Francisco: Harper & Row, 1981.

Young, John Z. *Programs of the Brain.* Oxford: Oxford University Press, 1978.

Readings on the Quantum Force

Bateson, Gregory. *Mind and Nature.* New York: E. P. Dutton, 1979.

Benson, Herbert. *The Mind/Body Effect.* New York: Simon & Schuster, 1979.

Blakeslee, Thomas R. *The Right Brain.* New York: Doubleday, 1980.

Budzynski, Thomas H. Tuning In on the "Twilight Zone." *Psychology Today,* 11 (1977), pp. 38–44.

Ferguson, Marilyn. *The Aquarian Conspiracy.* Los Angeles: J. P. Tarcher, 1980.

Gardiner, John W. *Excellence: Can We Be Equal and Excellent Too?* New York: Harper & Row (Perennial Library), 1971.

Hoffer, Eric. *The True Believer.* New York: Harper & Row (Perennial Library), 1966.

Lozanov, Georgi. *Suggestology and Outlines of Suggestopedy.* New York: Gordon and Breach, 1978.

Maltz, Maxwell. *Psycho-Cybernetics: The New Way to a Successful Life.* Englewood Cliffs, NJ: Prentice-Hall, 1960.

Maslow, Abraham H. *The Farther Reaches of Human Nature.* New York: Viking, 1971.

Nightingale, Earl. *This Is Earl Nightingale.* New York: Doubleday, 1969.

Ostrander, Sheila and Schroeder, Lynn et al. *Superlearning.* New York: Dell, 1979.

Selye, Hans. *Stress without Distress.* Philadelphia: J. B. Lippincott, 1974.

Stern, Aaron. *Me: The Narcissistic American.* New York: Ballantine, 1979.

Tiger, Lionel. *Optimism: The Biology of Hope.* New York: Simon & Schuster, 1979.

Waitley, Denis. *Seeds of Greatness: The Ten Best-Kept Secrets of Total Success.* New York: Pocket Books, 1984.

Readings on Quantum Nutrition and Exercise

Appenzeller, Otto and Atkinson, Ruth. *Sports Medicine: Fitness, Training, Injuries.* Baltimore, MD: Urban and Schwarzenberg, 1983.

BIBLIOGRAPHY

Brody, Jane. *Jane Brody's Nutrition Book.* New York: Bantam, 1982.
Dominguez, Richard and Gajda, Robert. *Total Body Training.* New York: Scribner, 1982.
Gutin, Bernard. *The High Energy Factor.* New York: Random House, 1983.
Hamilton, Eva M. and Whitney, Eleanor N. *Nutrition, Concepts and Controversies.* St. Paul, MN: West, 1982.
Katch, Frank I. and McArdle, William D. *Nutrition, Weight Control, and Exercise.* Philadelphia: Lea and Febiger, 1983.
Martin, Robert M. *A Clinical View of the Gravity Guidance System* (unpublished).
Remington, Dennis W., Fisher, Garth A. and Parent, Edward A. *How to Lower Your Fat Thermostat.* Provo, UT: Vitality House International, 1983.

APPENDIX A

Dietary Fiber in Your Food

Food	Serving Size	Weight (g)	Fiber (g)
Breads and Crackers			
Graham crackers	2 squares	15	1.5
Rye bread	1 slice	25	2.0
Rye crackers	3 wafers	20	2.3
Whole-wheat bread	1 slice	25	2.4
Cereals			
All-Bran or 100% Bran	1 cup	70	23.0
Bran Buds	¾ cup	60	18.0
Cracked wheat (bulgur), dry	⅓ cup	50	5.6
Grape-Nuts	⅓ cup	45	5.0
Grits, dry	¼ cup	45	4.8
Rolled oats, dry	½ cup	60	4.5
Shredded wheat	2 biscuits	50	6.1
Fruits			
Apple	1 small	90	3.1
Applesauce	½ cup	120	1.7
Banana	1 medium	100	1.8
Cantaloupe, cubes	¾ cup	120	1.4
Cherries, raw	10	70	0.8
Grapefruit	½	200	2.6
Grapes, raw	16	60	0.4
Orange	1 small	90	1.8
Peach, raw	1 medium	100	1.3
Peaches, canned slices	½ cup	120	1.3
Pear, raw	1 medium	120	2.8
Pears, canned	½ cup	125	1.4
Plum, raw	2 small	90	1.6
Strawberries	½ cup	125	2.6
Tangerine	1 medium	100	2.1

Food	Serving Size	Weight (g)	Fiber (g)
Vegetables			
Beans, green	½ cup	50	1.2
Beets, cooked	⅔ cup	100	2.1
Broccoli, cooked	¾ cup	75	1.6
Cabbage, cooked	¾ cup	100	2.2
Cabbage, raw	1 cup	75	2.1
Carrots, cooked	¾ cup	100	2.1
Carrots, raw	1 medium	100	3.7
Cauliflower, cooked	½ cup	100	1.2
Cauliflower, raw	1 cup	100	1.8
Celery, cooked	⅔ cup	100	2.4
Celery, raw	2½ stalks	100	3.0
Corn kernels	⅔ cup	110	4.2
Cucumber	½ of 7-inch cucumber	100	1.5
Kale, cooked	½ cup	100	2.0
Kidney beans, cooked	1 cup	75	3.6
Lentils, cooked	½ cup	100	4.0
Lettuce	1 cup	50	0.8
Parsnips, cooked	¾ cup	120	5.9
Peas, cooked	½ cup	60	3.8
Potatoes, cooked	⅔ cup	90 (raw)	3.1
Rice, brown, cooked	1 cup	65	1.1
Rice, white, cooked	1 cup	65	0.4
Spinach	2 large leaves	50	1.8
Summer squash, cooked	½ cup	100	2.2
Summer squash, raw	1 5-inch squash	100	3.0
Turnips, raw	1 cup	100	2.2

Source: The above fiber analyses were prepared by Dr. James W. Anderson, professor of medicine and clinical nutrition at the University of Kentucky Medical Center in Lexington, Kentucky.

APPENDIX B

Protein in "Protein" Foods

Food	Serving Size	Grams Protein
Bacon	2 medium slices	3.8
Beef, chuck roast	3 ounces cooked	24.0
Beef, lean ground	¼ pound raw	23.4
Bologna	3 slices (3 ounces)	10.2
Cheese, American	1 ounce slice	6.6
Cheese, cheddar	1 ounce	7.1
Cheese, cottage	½ cup	15.0
Chicken, fryer	1 drumstick	12.2
Eggs	2 medium	11.4
Fish sticks	3 sticks (3 ounces)	14.1
Flounder	3 ounces	25.5
Frankfurter	1 (2 ounces)	7.1
Ham, boiled	3 slices (3 ounces)	16.2
Kidney, beef	½ cup cooked	23.1
Lamb, rib chop	3 ounces	17.9
Liver, chicken	1 liver	6.6
Mackerel	3 ounces	18.6
Milk, skim	1 cup	8.8
Peanut butter	2 tablespoons	8.0
Pizza, cheese	¼ 14-inch pie	15.6
Pork, loin	3 ounces	20.8
Pork sausage	2 links (2 ounces)	5.4
Scallops	3 ounces friend	16.0
Shrimp	3 ounces fried	11.6
Tuna, canned	3 ounces drained	24.4
Turkey	3 ounces	26.8
Veal, stew meat	3 ounces	23.7
Yogurt	1 cup	8.3

APPENDIX C

Protein in Other Foods

Food	Serving Size	Grams Protein
Banana	1 medium	1.3
Barley	¼ cup raw	4.1
Bean curd (tofu)	1 piece	9.4
Beans, kidney	½ cup cooked	7.2
Beans, lima	½ cup cooked	6.5
Beans, navy	½ cup cooked	7.4
Bean sprouts (mung)	½ cup	2.0
Bran flakes (40%)	1 cup	3.6
Bread, rye	1 slice	2.3
Bread, white	1 slice	2.4
Bread, whole wheat	1 slice	2.6
Broccoli	½ cup	2.4
Bulgur	1 cup cooked	8.4
Corn	½ cup kernels	2.7
Farina	1 cup cooked in water	3.2
Lentils	½ cup cooked	7.8
Macaroni	1 cup cooked	6.5
Muffin, corn	1 medium	2.8
Noodles, egg	1 cup cooked	6.6
Oatmeal	1 cup cooked in water	4.8
Pancakes	3 4-inch cakes	5.7
Peas, green	½ cup cooked	4.3
Potato	7 ounces baked	4.0
Rice, brown	1 cup cooked	4.9
Rice, white	1 cup cooked	4.1
Sesame seeds	1 tablespoon	1.5
Soup, bean with pork	1 cup with water	8.0
Soup, chicken noodle	1 cup with water	3.4
Soup, cream of mushroom	1 cup with milk	6.9

Food	Serving Size	Grams Protein
Soup, tomato	1 cup with milk	6.5
Soup, vegetable	1 cup with water	2.2
Soybeans	½ cup cooked	9.9
Spaghetti	1 cup cooked al dente	6.5
Squash, acorn	1 cup baked	3.9
Sweet potato	5 ounces baked	2.4
Walnuts	10 large	7.3
Wheat flakes	1 cup	3.1
Wheat, shredded	2 biscuits	5.0

FAT-CHOLESTEROL CHART

Dairy Products and Related Products

	Serving Size	Total Fat (grams)	Saturated Fatty Acids (grams)	Monounsaturated Fatty Acids (grams)	Polyunsaturated Fatty Acids (grams)	Cholesterol (milligrams)	Food Energy (calories)
Milk:							
Fluid Whole	1 cup	8.2	5.1	2.4	0.3	33	125
2% (nonfat milk solids added)	1 cup	4.7	2.9	1.4	0.2	18	125
1%	1 cup	2.6	1.6	0.8	0.1	10	102
Skim	1 cup	0.4	0.3	0.1	Trace	4	86
Buttermilk (cultured)	1 cup	2.2	1.3	0.6	0.1	9	99
Cheese:							
American (Pasteurized Process)	1 oz.	8.9	5.6	2.5	0.3	27	106
Blue	1 oz.	8.2	5.3	2.2	0.2	21	100
Camembert	1⅓ oz.	9.2	5.8	2.7	0.3	27	114
Cheddar	1 oz.	9.4	6.0	2.7	0.3	30	114
Cottage—Creamed (4% fat)	1 cup	9.5	6.0	2.7	0.3	31	217
Cottage—Uncreamed (1% fat)	1 cup	2.3	1.5	0.7	0.1	10	164
Cream	1 Tbsp.	4.9	3.1	1.4	0.2	15	49

Feta	1 oz.	6.0	4.2	1.3	0.2	25	75
Mozzarella (made from partially skimmed milk)	1 oz.	4.5	2.9	1.3	0.1	16	72
Muenster	1 oz.	8.5	5.4	2.5	0.2	27	104
Parmesan	1 Tbsp.	1.5	1.0	0.4	Trace	4	23
Port du Salut	1 oz.	8.0	4.7	2.6	0.2	35	100
Ricotta (part skim)	1 oz.	2.2	1.4	0.7	0.1	9	39
Roquefort	1 oz.	8.7	0.5	2.4	0.4	26	105
Swiss	1 oz.	7.8	5.0	2.1	0.3	26	107
Tilsit (whole milk)	1 oz.	7.4	4.8	2.0	0.2	29	96
Cream:							
Light	1 Tbsp.	2.9	1.8	0.8	0.1	10	29
Heavy Whipping (unwhipped)	1 Tbsp.	5.6	3.5	1.6	0.2	21	52
Sour (cultured)	1 Tbsp.	2.5	1.6	0.7	0.1	5	26
Imitation cream products made with vegetable fat:							
Liquid	1 Tbsp.	1.5	1.4	Trace	Trace	0	20
Powdered	1 Tbsp.	2.1	1.8	Trace	Trace	0	33
Related Products:							
Ice Milk (soft serve)	1 cup	4.6	2.9	1.3	0.2	13	223
Ice Milk (hardened)	1 cup	5.7	3.6	1.7	0.2	18	184
Ice Cream—Reg. (approx 10% fat)	1 cup	14.3	8.9	4.1	0.5	59	269
Yogurt (plain made from partially skimmed milk)	8 oz. (1 cup)	3.5	2.3	1.0	0.1	14	144

Fats and Oils

	Size Serving	Total Fat (grams)	Saturated Fatty Acids (grams)	Monounsaturated Fatty Acids (grams)	Polyunsaturated Fatty Acids (grams)	Cholesterol (milligrams)	Food Energy (calories)
Peanut Butter	2 Tbsp.	16.0	3.0	7.4	4.6	0	190
Bacon (cooked crisp)	2 slices	8.0	2.5	3.7	0.7	14	85
Bacon Canadian (unheated)	3¼ oz.	14.4	4.9	6.6	1.5	75	216
Butter	1 Tbsp.	11.4	7.1	3.3	0.4	31	100
Lard	1 Tbsp	13.0	5.1	5.3	1.3	13	115
Tub Margarines:							
Safflower oil, liquid[1,2]	1 Tbsp.	11.4	1.6	2.6	6.7	0	101
Corn oil, liquid[1,2]	1 Tbsp.	11.4	2.0	4.5	4.4	0	102
Stick Margarines							
Corn oil, liquid[1,2]	1 Tbsp.	11.4	2.5	4.4	3.9	0	102
Stick or Tub Margarines Partially hydrogenated or hardened fat[1,2]	1 Tbsp.	11.4	2.2	4.9	3.7	0	102
Imitation Margarine (Diet)[2]	1 Tbsp.	5.5	1.1	2.2	2.0	0	49
Mayonnaise	1 Tbsp.	11.0	2.0	2.4	5.6	8	100
Vegetable Shortening (hydrogenated)	1 Tbsp.	13.0	3.2	5.7	3.1	0	110

	Amount						
Canned fish:							
Sardines (canned in oil; drained solids)	3¼ oz. (1 can)	9.0	3.0	2.5	0.5	129	175
Salmon, pink (canned)	3 oz	5.0	1.3	1.2	0.1	32	120
Tuna (packed in oil, drained solids)	3 oz.	7.0	1.7	1.4	1.4	55	167
Related Products:							
Liver, beef	3 oz.	9.0	2.5	3.5	0.9	372	195
Sweetbreads, calf	3 oz.	1.8	No Data	No Data	No Data	396	82
Frankfurters, (all beef—30% fat) 8 per lb.	1	16.3	6.6	8.2	0.7	49	170
Eggs (chicken, whole)	1 medium	5.6	1.7	2.2	0.7	274	79

Cooked Meat, Poultry, Fish and Related Products

	Size Serving	Total Fat (grams)	Saturated Fatty Acids (grams)	Monounsaturated Fatty Acids (grams)	Polyunsaturated Fatty Acids (grams)	Cholesterol (milligrams)	Food Energy (calories)
Lean Beef	3 oz.	7.7	3.7	3.4	0.2	77	177
Lean Pork and Ham	3 oz.	9.3	3.4	3.9	0.8	76	186
Lean Lamb	3 oz.	6.2	3.5	2.2	0.1	85	140
Lean Veal	3 oz.	5.1	2.5	2.4	.08	84	174
Poultry (flesh without skin):							
Light meat	3 oz.	4.2	1.3	1.5	0.8	74	155
Dark meat	3 oz.	5.5	1.7	2.1	1.0	74	157
Fish							
Lean	3 oz.	0.5	.08	.07	0.18	43	115
Fat	3 oz.	5.4	1.0	1.6	2.2	40	138
Shellfish:							
Crab	½ cup	2.0	0.5	0.7	0.8	62	85
Clams	6 large	1.0	0.3	0.3	0.4	36	65
Lobster	½ cup	1.0	0.1	0.2	0.4	62	68
Oysters	3 oz. (6 oysters)	1.5	0.5	0.2	0.8	45	90
Shrimp	½ cup (11 large)	1.0	0.2	0.3	0.5	96	100

Polyunsaturated Oils:

Corn Oil	1 Tbsp.	14.0	1.7	3.3	7.8	0	120
Cottonseed Oil	1 Tbsp.	14.0	3.7	2.6	7.1	0	120
Safflower Oil	1 Tbsp.	14.0	1.5	1.6	10.0	0	120
Sesame Oil	1 Tbsp.	14.0	2.1	5.5	5.7	0	120
Soybean Oil	1 Tbsp.	14.0	2.1	3.2	8.1	0	120
Soybean Oil (lightly hydrogenated)	1 Tbsp.	14.0	2.0	5.8	4.7	0	120
Sunflower Oil	1 Tbsp.	14.0	1.5	2.9	8.9	0	120

Monounsaturated Oils:

Olive Oil	1 Tbsp.	14.0	1.9	9.7	1.1	0	120
Peanut Oil	1 Tbsp.	14.0	2.3	6.2	4.2	0	120

Saturated Oil:

Coconut Oil	1 Tbsp.	14.0	12.1	0.8	0.3	0	120

[1] First ingredient as listed on label.
[2] Summary of available data. Composition of margarine changes periodically.